YOGA OF THE HEART

Yoga of the Heart

A WHITE EAGLE BOOK OF YOGA

Jenny Beeken

THE WHITE EAGLE PUBLISHING TRUST
NEW LANDS · LISS · HAMPSHIRE · ENGLAND

First published May 1990

© Jenny Beeken, 1990
Illustrations © Andrew Slocock, 1990

British Library Cataloguing in Publication Data
Beeken, Jenny, *1948—*
Yoga of the heart.
1. Iyengar yoga
I. Title
613.7

ISBN 0-85487-080-6

Set in 10 on 12pt Bodoni and
printed in Great Britain by
William Clowes Ltd, London and Beccles

Contents

---------------- **PART ONE** ----------------

PART TWO

Preface

by JOAN HODGSON

JENNY BEEKEN has been giving me yoga lessons since the spring of 1981 and I can truly say that her method of teaching has been of the greatest possible help. Since my early twenties I had suffered intermittently with back trouble and sciatica which, on many occasions, necessitated quite a long rest in bed. Since I started working with Jenny, and faithfully performed the postures and movements she gave me, there has been no return of the trouble at all.

Jenny attended several of B. K. S. Iyengar's training courses, both in India and in Britain, and gained his intermediate certificate. To attain this specialized and advanced qualification required constant work and practice, both in teaching and performance, and her lessons help me to realize ever more clearly the true meaning of 'yoga', which is union: union of our whole being with the Great White Spirit and with all life, in nature and in our fellow beings. This realization dawns gently and slowly as, through patient practice of the postures, the whole body seems to become more alive—I would almost say 'more aware', in every cell, of an inflow of divine energy.

This comes not through any forcing or violent stretching, for we are taught that there should never be any strain in yoga, or any forcing of the body into unnatural positions by the will and domination of the outer mind. The control seems to come from a quiet inner command, the will of the spirit, which is gentle yet firm.

Since Jenny produced her practice cassettes, I have found it most helpful to work with them, following exactly her gentle instructions which are particularly helpful to use on the days when the body lazily resists being brought into action. Somehow then the sound of her voice pulls one gently up into *tadasana*, the Mountain pose ... and so on, into the others. Almost immediately there comes a feeling of the sun shining down above one's head and the strength and steadiness of mother earth beneath one's feet, the energy flowing through one's whole being with every breath.

White Eagle tells us:

Our brother Indians were perfect physically, and spiritually much in advance of the white man today. Have you ever watched a Red Indian walking? You should take a lesson from that. Think for a moment of the difference in your attitude of mind immediately you pull yourself erect and aspire. You seem to be filled with light, and this is exactly what happens when you stand erect, perfectly poised. The spiritual light is able to enter and pass through you without hindrance, to your fingertips and down your spine to its base; and your feet (free and supple, as they should be) are able to feel and draw magnetism from the earth, and this magnetism circulates through your aura, giving you that vitality and energy for which you long.

It is most important to keep the spine straight, my children, so that the energy of the Sun spirit can pour through the head and descend down the spine. The body elemental is attached to the lower forms of life, it wants to slouch, but the ego wants to stand upright. An erect spine helps to keep the soul in touch with the higher self, rather than to remain under the influence of the body elemental. You can get a straight back as much from the mind as the body....

So few earthly brothers know how to relax. I see tense sleeping bodies, faces screwed up, instead of a beautiful relaxation, peace, and surrender to the heavenly spheres. When you go to bed at night, let your body rest at ease, your mind be calm and still, and let the celestial body fill the aura with the light of Christ.

In this way you will prepare yourself to go forth from your body into higher worlds; here you will undergo spiritual experiences which will so impress the mind that you will waken in the morning with a gentle memory of something wonderful having happened. In this preparation for sleep—and the way you sleep—you are training yourselves to receive divine illumination, and freedom from the chains of bondage of earthly life.

SUN-MEN OF THE AMERICAS

With regular practice, gradually the realization dawns that each posture, gently performed, with the mind focused peacefully on the task in hand, can be in itself a meditation, while the relaxation at the end brings an increasing awareness of the beauty of quiet breathing (*pranayama*), absorbing into every cell of one's being the divine breath. At first the outer mind tends to resist the relaxation/meditation after postures, almost regarding it as a nice extra, when time allows, rather than an essential part of practice.

It takes patience and time to come to this realization, but I can vouch for every statement Jenny makes in her book about yoga awakening the whole consciousness to the divine life. It is an awareness, subtle and all-pervasive, which dawns as we keep on keeping on steadily with the gentle practice. There comes a quickening appreciation of beauty in all its forms, but especially in nature; a growing awareness of the life-force in plants and trees, and almost a feeling of uniting with them in their growth.

There comes increased sympathy and awareness of divine life in animal and insect, and of course even more so in our fellow beings. Then in an even more subtle way this awareness extends to the angelic kingdom, until the brotherhood of all life becomes a living reality.

People have sometimes asked why we encourage yoga classes in an organisation which is orientated towards giving service on the inner planes through prayer and meditation and sending out the light, rather than towards physical culture. But I have learned through the practice of yoga that the body is truly an instrument of the spirit. Just as an artist can create more beautiful pictures or sculptures with adequate materials of good quality and the musician can produce better music on a perfect instrument, so in spiritual work the radiation of light and thought-power can be far more effective when a steady nervous system, a harmonious flexible body, and an understanding of breath control, can facilitate the inflow of divine energy.

Again, White Eagle confirms this:

One of the finest methods of which we knew in our American Indian days for the strengthening of the finer bodies and nervous system was by deep breathing. People little realize the importance of breathing correctly, and how the art of breathing can be used to cleanse and revivify not only the physical body but every part of man's being....

The Indian never hurried [his] morning communion with the Great White Spirit and the angels of the elements. It was an essential part of his life and one which never failed to bring renewed vitality and strength of purpose for the day's tasks which lay ahead. Deep breathing brings an inner tranquillity, a steadiness and valuable help in facing any ordeals which lie ahead. A master never allows himself to become flustered or worried; a master can face anything with perfect calm.

SUN-MEN OF THE AMERICAS

Practice of many of the yoga postures may seem too difficult for souls whose karma has given them a body disabled in some way, but everyone can practise and benefit from the method of breathing described by Jenny Beeken and practised in the White Eagle Lodge meditation classes. Also, there are simple relaxed positions which can be prescribed by a teacher to help almost any physical infirmity.

We are not suggesting that yoga is the only form of physical exercise which is valuable in spiritual unfoldment, but the disciplines originating in the East, such as T'ai Chi, are possibly more helpful than most western methods, which are geared almost entirely to physical training and take little account of spiritual unfoldment and soul harmony. It is of course perfectly possible to arrive at the same point in spiritual unfoldment by other means.

But over the years, in the White Eagle work, we have come to realize that discipline of the physical body through suitable exercise can greatly facilitate the unfoldment of the mental and spiritual powers.

I hope that this book, combined perhaps with Jenny's cassettes or video, will help many friends to discover the same benefits as I have experienced. I can truly say that my body now is more comfortable and flexible than when I was in my twenties and thirties! But once started, it is necessary just to keep on keeping on, to use White Eagle's time-honoured phrase, for you will discover that the benefits of yoga are cumulative, increasing as one quietly persists. There seems to be a subtle but very real magic in this ancient practice which I can fully recommend to all followers of the White Eagle teaching.

New Lands, Liss, 1989

Acknowledgments

I first thank my mother, Olive Beeken, for the deep love shown by her tireless typing of my original manuscript over nearly four years. She ploughed through my handwriting, undeterred by its illegibility. Also, I thank her for being her, and for her constant support of me even when she thinks I am being crazy!

My great thanks go to the artist, Andrew Slocock, who diligently worked on one draft after another of the cover and drawings and was undaunted even by the loss of the (supposed) final jacket design on a train! Thank you too to those who were responsible for putting the manuscript on the word-processor—to Aphra Peard, Ann Clarke, Nigel Millross and Chryssa Porter; and to those responsible for the many photographic and printing sessions—Bruce Clarke, Iris Oliver, Debbie Low, Anthony King, Pauline Sawyer, Colum and Jeremy Hayward.

I greatly appreciate the tremendous work done by my editors, Colum and Jeremy Hayward, in working on my grammar and phrasing, and thank them for their many, many hours of help and support on every level during the work on this book.

My great thanks also to Ylana Hayward and Joan Hodgson at the White Eagle Lodge for their love and support over the years, especially the last twelve months: their help and advice with the editing of the book and with my personal life—during my pregnancy and while I was giving birth almost simultaneously to my baby and this book; also to the rest of the family at New Lands, particularly Jenny Dent for her loving friendship, and 'Radiance' for her deep thoughtful help and love, first on earth and then from the spirit spheres.

My deep love, devotion and great gratitude go to Shri B.K.S. Iyengar for the great inspiration, vitality and love he showed to me. He truly 'woke me up' on my visits to Poona, India, and brought out my Inner Self, which had previously been under a dark cloud. I will always admire and respect his tremendous energy, dedication and enthusiasm for yoga, and his very astute perception of the body and its reflection of the Inner Self.

I thank Kofi Busia for originally introducing me to yoga at the level at which it is all-embracing, and for the great precision, perception and understanding that he brings to the teaching of the *asanas*. My deep thanks and love go to Angela Farmer and Victor Van Kooten for their inspired teaching of their own truth in yoga and in life, and in showing that the two are synonymous and that we can all find our own truth for ourselves. Also for the very great love and support that they both have given me.

I also give great thanks to Graham and Elizabeth Browne of the Bellin Partnership (formerly the Self-Transformation Centre) who, through their work, gave me a much greater understanding of the philosophy of yoga and how we can apply it and live it in the West. Their teaching and philosophy taught me how to live my life happily and contentedly and not to be afraid to be what I am.

Much love and thanks to Jill Moffitt and her family for the luxury stay in Connecticut, USA, which enabled me to spend time on this book, and to Jill for her inspirational help and advice with the manuscript.

Finally, my great thanks and gratitude to all those who have stepped in supportively to take my classes and have thus given me space and time to write this book, as well as on all the other occasions that I have needed time off; to June Elliott-Thomas, for her marvellous administrative and organisational support—a real friend; to Pauline Sawyer, for always being there when needed, especially with the photographs—again a real friend; and to Pip Cooper, Kirsty Dennis and (again) Jeremy Hayward.

And to all the many, many other pupils, friends and family who have lovingly supported me in my work and my life over the last ten years.

Jenny Beeken: Petersfield, 1989

Publishers' Acknowledgments

We wish to thank the following publishers, organizations and individuals for kind permission to use their copyright material in the text.

Fine Line Books Ltd, 5 Water Eaton Rd, Oxford OX2 7QQ for the paragraphs from THE TREE OF YOGA, © B. K. S. Iyengar, 1988. Self-Realization Fellowship, 3880 San Rafael Ave., Los Angeles, Calif. 90065, for the quotation from Paramahansa Yogananda's AUTOBIOGRAPHY OF A YOGI. Celestial Arts, P.O. Box 7327, Berkeley, Calif. 94707 for the sentences from LOVE IS LETTING GO OF FEAR © Gerald G. Jampolsky, 1979. Bantam Books for the quotations from EMMANUEL'S BOOK and EMMANUEL'S BOOK II, © Pat Rodegast, 1985 and 1989. Unwin Hyman Ltd for the four passages from THE UPANISHADS, except that on p. 15, in the translation © Alistair Shearer and Peter Russell, 1978; and for the quotation from LIGHT ON YOGA by B. K. S. Iyengar, © George Allen & Unwin (Publishers) Ltd, 1966, 1968, 1976. Faber and Faber for two quotations from THE GEETA: THE GOSPEL OF THE LORD SHREE KRISHNA, translated by Shree Purohit Swami, 1935. Harper & Row Publishers, Inc., for a sentence from KINSHIP WITH ALL LIFE, © J. Allen Boone, 1954. Penguin Books Ltd, 27 Wrights Lane, London W8 5TZ for the affirmation from A COURSE IN MIRACLES, © Foundation for Inner Peace, Inc., Tiburan, Calif., 1975, and the quotation on p. 15 from THE UPANISHADS, in the translation © Juan Mascaró, 1965. New World Library, San Rafael, Calif. 94913, for the affirmation excerpted from LIVING IN THE LIGHT by Shakti Gawain with Laurel King, © Shakti Gawain, 1986. The Krishnamurti Foundation Trust, Ltd., Brockwood Park Bramdean, Hampshire SL24 0LQ, for the extract from KRISHNAMURTI'S JOURNAL, © 1982. The New Book Society of India for the quotation from GLORIOUS THOUGHTS OF TAGORE, © 1965.

PART ONE

Yoga in the West

Who sees all beings in his own Self, and his own Self in all beings, loses all fear.
ISA UPANISHAD

THERE ARE MANY books which give instruction in how to practise the postures, the breathing, the mantras and the meditations of yoga, and others that give an excellent academic interpretation of the philosophy of yoga. My aim in this book is to help the reader experience yoga on all levels, without the separation that tends to exist in the West between the practice of the postures and the philosophy of yoga. We tend to compartmentalize in our minds: a compartment for the physical aspects and the breathing, a compartment for the spiritual aspects and meditation. For this reason the philosophy tends to attract the mind as a study, not as a way of living. And even though we are now beginning to see the wisdom in eastern ideas and use this philosophy in many areas (an example is the way the principle of complementarity clarifies the wave/particle theory in physics) we still find the aspect of yoga which is concerned with physical postures does not integrate easily with the aspect of yoga which is a philosophy and, when taken as an individual path, a religion.

This is why I have chosen to use the message of a Western spiritual teacher—White Eagle—in this book. In his words, perhaps uniquely, both the physical and the spiritual aspects of yoga seem to be completely at home.

Yoga, from the Sanskrit *yuj*, means union: that is, union of the little self on earth with the God-self, the Higher Self, the Divine spark within us. Yoga is a way of life, a path that is at least five thousand years old in India: it is all-inclusive, all-encompassing, and one with all religions. It is a path that takes the Self to God; it is ancient wisdom.

White Eagle too refers to his teachings as the ancient wisdom, a wisdom that has been with us for all time, that is timeless, all-knowing and deep within each one of us. It is there for us all if we should choose to look deep within ourselves. The ancient wisdom is there at the base of all religions and it is the source of all true spiritual teachings. It was evident in ancient Egypt, in the early North and South American Indian cultures and in esoteric Christianity, and it can be found throughout the teachings of the East, in the Tao and in Yoga.

White Eagle's teaching takes its framework from esoteric Christianity but he would say that these teachings are one with the teachings of yoga, and perhaps a look at the two will help us to bring more understanding to the use of yoga in the West. In his very helpful, down-to-earth advice about daily life (which nonetheless comes from deep spiritual wisdom), White Eagle refers to yoga in the light of the spirit, showing us how a deep spiritual awareness can be brought through the layers of consciousness to manifest as a way of living for us here in the West, caught up otherwise in crazily busy lives.

Over nearly twenty years I have absorbed and been helped and uplifted by the timeless wisdom of White Eagle; at the same time I have had the privilege of having B. K. S. Iyengar as a yoga teacher during my two visits to India and on his various visits to the West. Although I started to practise the postures, the breathing and the meditation from a physical and mental viewpoint, to give me a healthy body and a sound, steady mind, I have gradually realized over the years how the physical practice of yoga enables us to touch the spirit deep within. I now more fully understand some words of White Eagle's which I shall cite in a specific context later on:

The way to truth is through the spirit. In the outer world there is turmoil and chaos and unhappiness. You *think* with the mortal mind, with the mind which is part of the substance of earth. You should think with your inner mind, you should approach problems through the inner self, through intuition. The very word explains itself. In-tuition—training inside yourself. You are looking outside for help, and all the time the help you want is inside. The world of spirit that so many of you talk about and believe in, and long to touch, is all within.

THE QUIET MIND

I started practising yoga because I felt heavy, depressed, weighed down by the conditions of the world and the conditions of my own mind. I received healing from the White Eagle Lodge for the same reason and have found that gradually over the years the two have worked together for me, to help me understand the workings of the spirit within us that is at one with all life and is the source of our aliveness, our joy and love for ourselves and others. So although I started yoga from a more outward viewpoint and came to White Eagle's teaching to find an answer to personal problems, both have led me to understand the deep inner need within us for a spiritually-based life. The awareness of this life grows out of day-to-day practice of postures and affirmations, which together enable us to touch the spirit. This book gives help and advice for that daily practice.

I have met many people with misconceptions and fears about yoga. Some see it just as a system of strange physical postures designed to keep the body in a healthy, fit, relaxed condition. This it is, but such a view of yoga is a very limited one. Others regard it as a rather dangerous facet of Eastern religion. Yoga is actually a path to God, through self-knowing, self-understanding and self-discipline. The 'union' which the word implies represents a union on all levels: the union of the earthly self with the Higher Self, the union of soul with God, the union of the mind and body, the heart and spirit, the union of one soul to another—as well as the union of the self to mother earth and to all of nature. This to me is the meaning of yoga. Through its daily practice one begins to experience at-one-ment with all life. Life lived in oneness is life lived in yoga; thus it is not necessary to practise the postures to be practising yoga.

Both the path of yoga and the path described in White Eagle's teaching are heart-centred: that is, they teach that all our actions, thoughts and awareness need to come from the heart of our being. If they do, then we live and work from love and have our being in love. White Eagle calls this Christ-consciousness, and the aim of his teaching is to bring Christ-consciousness to the heart of humanity, Jesus Christ being the most perfect example here on earth of Christ-consciousness manifesting in man.

The path of yoga recognizes this same Christ-consciousness, although it is not immediately apparent that it does. Hinduism encompasses many aspects of God and people misinterpret this to mean many gods, but the pictorial representation and images of the different aspects are used to help us to make contact with and understand all the facets. For example, Ganesha, the god of wisdom, helps us to understand the wisdom aspect. Christ-consciousness represents perfected consciousness, all the various facets of the jewel polished and perfected. All the yogis of the East with whom I have come into contact, either in person or through the written word, have pointed to the dawn of the Christ-consciousness today in a world that greatly needs it. Thus, in AUTOBIOGRAPHY OF A YOGI, Paramahansa Yogananda writes:

Yoga is a method for restraining the natural turbulence of thoughts, which otherwise impartially prevents all men, of all lands, from glimpsing their true nature of Spirit. Like the healing light of the sun, yoga is beneficial equally to men of the East and men of the West. The thoughts of most persons are restless and capricious; a manifest need exists for yoga, the science of mind control.... There are a number of great men, living today in American or European or other non-Hindu bodies, who, though they may never have heard the words *yogi* and *swami*, are yet true exemplars of those terms. Through their disinterested service to mankind, or through their mastery over passions and thoughts, or through their singlehearted love of God, or through their great powers of concentration, they are, in a sense, yogis.

And White Eagle says:

Yoga means a state of union between the little self and the spirit. A yogi is not necessarily an Easterner, but one who has attained complete union with God. Jesus Christ was the greatest yogi. The form of Jesus when he demonstrated that great truth to humanity was the ever-beautiful body of a young man. The form gets to that perfect state and remains. One belongs, one is part, one is whole and one henceforth lives in that consciousness—individualized, yes, but consciously united. That soul is called thereafter by that simple word, so misunderstood in the western world, a yogi. A yogi is one who has found at-one-ment or union with the whole, with the universe. When that one has reached the apex of life, he only knows the way to live in love: he loves everything, everybody, every creature; he cannot do other than love. God is love, and when a man has attained love he has attained all.

The latter quotation particularly demonstrates to me the oneness between yoga and White Eagle's teaching. When,

throughout this book, I have stated that yoga has this or that effect, for me this is synonymous with following White Eagle's teaching. Similarly, in stating the effects of yoga, I am not exclusively referring to the postures, but to the whole way of life which incorporates the philosophy and the meditational technique of yoga. The path that we think of as yoga is not necessarily right for everyone. Yet I hope that even if you do not consider yourself a yoga practitioner you will still be interested in reading this book, since once you are aware of the principles of yoga you will realize that many people are already practising them—possibly unconsciously—just by the way that they naturally live their lives, in a state of near-oneness with all life and with God.

As I have said, the way of meditation given in most yoga teachings, as well as that given by White Eagle, is heart-centred. The whole awareness and concentration is centred in the heart. Meditation, whatever the method that is used, is a way of going to the source—not an end in itself. The aim of meditation is union of the self with God.

There are some techniques of meditation that concentrate on drawing energy up from the base centres. Such techniques can be dangerous if they are indulged in before the soul is ready and strong enough to cope with the extra energy that is being generated. There are also brow-centred meditations that stimulate a lot of power in the individual, which again is potentially explosive. However, if the meditation is heart-centred this can only stimulate love through unity—the essence of White Eagle's teachings and the essence of yoga.*

It is very easy to take from any ancient source of teaching just what we want to hear as a means of comfort to our outer self, instead of listening to our hearts for the meaning. The heart says that growth comes through taking up the challenge to live life in wholeness. White Eagle links yoga to a life lived consciously, thoughtfully, in close communion with the natural world. A book

*See the book list at the end for the White Eagle books on meditation.

that I shall quote from time to time, SUN-MEN OF THE AMERICAS (written by his medium, Grace Cooke, but with many of his original words), is about the North American Indians but has much in it that is pure yoga. He encourages us to stand firm and straight on the earth, to be centred in our hearts; to quieten our busy minds, to discipline ourselves, our bodies, through breathing, posture and meditation; so that we are able to live happy, contented lives on earth in service to humanity, and yet be one with our spirit within and the spirit within all that is around us in all humanity, in the earth, in the animal, plant and mineral kingdoms and in the whole of the cosmos. Yoga is a way of working towards and achieving this heart-centred awareness of the spirit within ourselves and in all life.

I have avoided intellectual comparisons in writing this book, so that I can express the symbolic and inner effects of the postures, breathing exercises and meditations of yoga, and in the hope that their sacredness will be felt and used as prayers and rituals to bring about the oneness of life in its totality. I have used many White Eagle quotations as well as quotations from other sources to illumine and clarify the philosophy of yoga, which on first appearance may be challenging for the Westerner to grasp; and further, to illustrate the oneness of all ancient teachings. I hope this book may contribute to your understanding of the deeper significance of the practice of yoga, and that it can help you, as yoga has helped me, to live your life in wholeness.

Why Practise Yoga?

It behoves all of us, when we realize the truth that the body is indeed the temple of the spirit, to keep our bodies unsullied; to treat them with the same courtesy and gentleness with which God Himself regards them.

Remember, my sons and daughters, that your body is the temple of God and should be used with thankfulness to glorify God....

Keep your body pure and healthy; do not allow it to be overstrained; eat wisely, of pure food, and each day open yourself to the blessing of the Christ spirit, that your body may be illumined by the Son of God. So will you meet your fellow men with a blessing radiating from your heart; your hands will possess the power to heal, your words to comfort those in trouble; and your very aura will show forth the radiance of the Christ spirit, so that every soul you encounter may feel better for having come into touch with you.

White Eagle, in SUN-MEN OF THE AMERICAS, by Grace Cooke

The body is the temple of the spirit, and needs to be kept in a healthy condition in order for the spirit to shine through it into the life. The continued practice of yoga in all its aspects is one way of bringing about a healthy body, a healthy mind, a healthy emotional state of being. It keeps us in touch with our true self, the God within. It is often quite noticeable—with regular practice

from the beginning—that there is a sense of well-being, of ease in the physical body and the emotions.

This sense of well-being brings great joy and pleasure in actually doing the postures—the feeling of extending the body also extends the mind and releases pent-up emotions, so as to make one feel good on all levels. The discovery that you can go a little further and break barriers that you never thought you would brings a great sense of lightness and achievement, for through yoga anything is possible. White Eagle also says that everything is possible: it is only our minds that put a limit on things. This is true of the body: our minds and emotions have created our aches, stiffness, tension and dis-ease; and so through extending our bodies, trusting the body to know exactly how far we can go at any one point, we can break through tremendous barriers in our mind and unruly emotions. This brings a great sense of being master of our outer earthly selves, and a great sense of joy at that heavenly contact which comes through feeling our bodies uplifted, opened out, free of earthly heaviness.

On the way to this state of well-being there may be other more immediate effects, depending on the way yoga is approached and practised. It has been likened to a journey backwards through our life, and maybe it even touches on other lives, for the body has a memory of its own. In a way that is ultimately very useful, yoga can bring to the surface traumas, shocks and hurt that have been held in the body over a long time, or it can awaken pleasant memories and sensations, whether they are at a physical level or an emotional and psychological level. For instance, I have taught several people who have had physical accidents to their body, such as a whiplash to the neck in a car accident which has left the neck weak and vulnerable. In this state of vulnerability, most of us, like them, then protect this area by tightening all the surrounding muscles and ligaments across the shoulders and the upper back; and yet this reaction and holding-in, necessary as it feels at the time, actually holds in the trauma of that accident, maintaining a weakness there, creating a tightening, an armouring, all around that area. When we begin to stimulate this area through the practice of the postures, it may initially bring out a lot of the feeling that came as a result of the accident both as local pain and in the mind and emotions. This would be the point at which many people would say 'yoga is not for me, because I have this problem', and stop doing it—thereby still holding on to the past and past experience. But with the help of a skilful loving teacher they can instead be taken gently through that point by working the neck in such a way that it strengthens it and brings it back to life, using postures such as a Head-stand between two chairs, never taking weight on the head if the neck is weak; Shoulder-stand on blocks (all as described in the inverted posture section, chapter 8), Bridge pose (Backward bends, chapter 7); and simultaneously working to release the upper back and shoulder-muscles in the standing postures so that the whole area opens up and frees itself, thereby releasing the past.

The therapeutic effects of yoga take place on many levels, and in many ways. Some of the initial reactions to the postures can be dizziness, nausea, and discomfort in certain areas, or disturbing memories. This does not happen with everybody, but I have known many instances of such reactions, and it actually means that the yoga practice is really working to release the whole system from its past. If we can let go of any fear, let go of any tendency to wrap ourselves in the past, and just trust God and the natural ability of our body to bring us through, then after a relatively short time we shall completely release this tension; the strain that is held in the muscles, ligaments, organs, and bones of the body will disappear; and we shall feel that health and lightness which the practice of yoga ultimately brings.

Some of the effects of yoga can be very much at a psychological or an emotional level. For example, I have taught women who had miscarriages, had difficulties in childbirth or have been sexually abused; and these memories and associated feelings can be brought to the surface through yoga, an effect which often comes about with other natural forms of healing such as homeopathy. This is quite safe and part of the healing process, but it might be helpful in such a case to seek counselling help or to discuss the matter with the yoga teacher. Affirmations are very helpful— these are described in the *yamas* and the *niyamas* section. Massage and acupuncture can also help. The individual must choose the therapy he or she feels drawn to; but often the whole condition can be worked on just through *hatha* yoga. I find that it is on residential weeks and weekends particularly that these effects manifest, probably because people are out of their normal day-to-day environment and are able to 'let go' a little more; and also because they are in a loving group of people to whom they can turn for support and help. On my own courses we then work together in discussions and meditations and may use massage, Bach Flower Remedies, and so on, and be available to help one another through any difficulties. It is a good rule of thumb that it takes a month of constant yoga practice to release something which has been held onto for a year, rather like the time it takes a person to release the effects of smoking after they have given it up.

Some people come to these deeper effects of yoga when, after a couple of years of practice, they are about to stop doing it, thinking they have done yoga now and know what it's about. In fact it is just beginning to touch them at a deeper level, and by ceasing their practice, they are resisting going in that deeply. We all have the choice to do this, but we also have the choice to live in the present, not caught up in the effects of the past, and thus to be free and whole. Through yoga, and the knowledge that comes through yoga that there is nothing to fear at all, we can comparatively quickly release ourselves from the past.

Because of the inner release that the practice of yoga brings about, it has a very deep therapeutic effect on both physical and psychological levels. Yet at many points in the instructions to the postures given in this book, you will find that I say that if you have a certain problem, such as high blood pressure, the way you practise the postures can be modified to your particular need. These modifications are not to restrict you, or to say that you will never be able to do the postures completely, but are given in order to restore normality in the system first. I have, for instance, brought my own blood-pressure up to normal when it has dropped very low, by the practice of inverted postures. So do not think you will never be able to practise the postures fully if you are needing to work at the therapeutic level, for all yoga is therapy at some level, and everything changes over time. Take careful note of the cautions and modifications to the postures if they apply to you, as they are given very deliberately.

By using yoga in this way it is possible to do anything, cure anything, relieve any problem you may have, at whatever level. But it may be necessary to find a teacher who has experience in dealing with yoga as therapy, and who can tell intuitively how best to help you. If you have any difficulties finding a suitable teacher, please write to me at the New Lands address of the White Eagle Lodge.

Always remember that in all aspects of yoga, from the deepest meditation down to the simplest posture, the aim and ultimate effect is one-ness, unity, at-one-ment on all levels; and all the immediate effects that practice brings about are part of the path to that oneness. The simplest posture can very easily be the deepest meditation.

CHAPTER ONE

The Eight Limbs of Yoga

Have you ever thought what forgiveness means? You, your own self, your own personality, needs your forgiveness. Your spirit is divine, but until you have overcome, your personality remains human and needs the forgiveness of your spirit. As you forgive, as your spirit forgives your personality, so also you will learn to forgive your brother man for all his seeming errors. If you will train yourself to think in terms of love and forgiveness every moment of your life, a most beautiful healing will take place in you.

White Eagle, THE QUIET MIND

THE EIGHT LIMBS, as they are traditionally known, are an outline of the practice of the path of yoga. They are called limbs because it is not intended that we start at one and work sequentially through; rather, the practice of one brings about the practice of the others. The first two, the *yamas* and *niyamas*, are of crucial importance, for they refer to our relationships with others and how we live our life in the world, and if we were to practise the other six, which are the inner disciplines of posture (*asanas*), breathing (*pranayama*), and control of the senses (*pratyahara*), and the three stages of meditation (*dharana, dhyana* and *samadhi*), without regard to how we relate to those around us, we would not be able to fulfil our purpose here on earth.

Conversely, the remaining six limbs enable us to practise the first two limbs—the *yamas* and the *niyamas*. Indeed constant practice of the inner disciplines gradually, subtly, brings about the practice of the outer disciplines towards others, often without a conscious realization of the change within us. Others will often notice and remark on it before we ourselves are aware of it. In writing about the *yamas* and *niyamas* I have tried to show how the practice of physical postures helps to remove the obstacles which prevent us achieving the ideals that the *yamas* and *niyamas* set.

I. *Yamas*

The *yamas* are the ethical disciplines which help us to look at our life with regard to others. The practice of all the eight limbs enables us to change and work on ourselves in our interaction with our brothers and sisters on the earth. These *yamas* and *niyamas* may seem impossible for us to achieve when we look at our seeming faults, and judge the state of our minds and the world around us. So, to help, I have given affirmations at the end of each section which can further the understanding and the practice of the *yamas* and the *niyamas*. Positive affirmations are a way in which we can recondition our negative thoughts. We have many negative assertions constantly speaking to us like old records going round and round inside our heads. These negative

— 21 —

thought-patterns may come from things we have been told from early in our childhood, things that we have misinterpreted or taken too literally; things that are the unconscious prejudices of the time in which we live, and are picked up by us from the atmosphere around us, as well as from our parents, teachers, and from all those with whom we come into close contact. Little children, before the change of teeth, are extraordinarily receptive to thought-vibration. Most importantly, they feel the inner love and wisdom of the heart that flows from one person to another as well, but this can gradually become veiled by those outer fears and beliefs that become imprinted on the consciousness.

This is not a wholly bad thing. In fact, it is a necessary process, one which we as souls have chosen, before coming into incarnation, in order to work out our karma: a way in which we can have the experiences of limitation which we must have in order to grow. We choose both the lessons we should like to go through and the relationships with others which will give us the experiences we need. Creating this network of relationships, we give ourselves and others the impetus needed to develop the light within.

One of the things many of us were once encouraged to believe was that we are all sinners, even that we were born in sin. Little children today are sometimes told that they are naughty, wicked through and through, before they have any concept of what this means or any idea that what they are doing is considered 'wrong' in society. Most of this conditioning is completed before we are three years old and it stays with us, until we recognize it for what it is. If we take an objective look at our minds we can see how many injunctions we place on ourselves: that we are unworthy, for instance; that we are unlovable, that we can't succeed, that we are bad. Observe what you say to yourself when you feel frustrated and angry, when you have not matched up to your own expectations of yourself or those of others—the phrases you use can be most revealing! Such habits of thought can apply just as much on the spiritual path, when we tell ourselves that we cannot meditate, we are not peaceful, that we are no good because we

have angry, critical thoughts or impatient desires.

This is not to say that we do not need to set ourselves a 'marker at the end of the furrow', as White Eagle puts it, and aim towards it; but neither is it wise to be too hard on ourselves if we do not meet our own expectations, as this just results in feelings of guilt that are of no help to anyone. We do not need to judge ourselves, or indeed anyone else, in this way.

Jesus said, 'Judge not, that ye be not judged'. If we judge others are we not really judging ourselves, inasmuch as we see ourselves in other beings reflected as in a mirror? We surely deserve the same respect from ourselves as we give to others (and, indeed, as we expect from others). Are we not all connected, all part of the same whole? So we need to love ourselves, letting go of judgment; and in so doing we are creating a way by which we can in truth love others. The key here is acceptance, acceptance of ourselves and of others exactly as they are and as we are. Wanting to change others is only a lack of acceptance in ourselves of the things that others mirror for us: the things that irritate and upset us. From acceptance there comes a letting-go of what we no longer want or need in our lives, in our consciousness: things like competitiveness, or the need to prove ourselves. We do not need to be run by our negative self-image. We are much more, much greater than that in the true light of our spirit.

In creating positive affirmations we can recondition the outer mind to believe what the heart knows to be true. White Eagle gives us the most beautiful affirmations in PRAYER IN THE NEW AGE:

I AM Divine Love
I AM Divine Peace
I AM Divine Wisdom
I AM Divine Power

These are very powerful, evocative words. The 'I AM' is parallel to the Sanskrit 'Om'—the word which brings life into being; the same 'word' as St John used when he wrote: 'In the beginning was the Word'. Both the 'I am' and the 'Om' are powerful mantras and affirmations in themselves, stirring the divine life-force within us that brought us into being.

A mantra is a syllable or series of syllables that strikes a note deep within us, clearing all that is in the way of our touching the Source. It is the vibration a mantra creates rather than the meaning of the mantra that is most important and effective. So the affirmation 'I am divine love' brings out that deep divine love within the heart that brings oneness and unity.

It is often recommended when using mantras to include your own name, to make them more effective for you. This splits up the 'I AM' into (say) 'I, Jenny, am divine love'. This can help to bring the divinity to every level of our being—through the personality to the mind and to the body. It ties in with the purpose of the practice of the postures of yoga, which is to bring the divine, the Higher Self, into every cell of the physical body, so that every cell is filled with divine love, divine peace, divine wisdom, divine power. However, to call upon the 'I AM' is to call upon the eternal spirit and holds a power all of its own. Therefore I find it most helpful to start without my name in order to stimulate the divine in the heart, and after repeating this to myself to bring in my own name and see the divine energy spreading to every cell. If you prefer not to split the 'I AM' you are not diminishing the effectiveness of the affirmation, but in many of the more detailed affirmations given in this section it is appropriate to make them personal.

This intensive work on ourselves may appear to some to be very introspective, but we live our lives more effectively in the world when we recognize and transform the patterns that veil the divinity within ourselves.

The affirmations given in the next section are specifically to help in the practice of the *yamas* and *niyamas*, especially if the principle brings up the feeling of difficulty and the fear that you cannot achieve it.

Affirmations can also work in a way that I have described in the section, 'Why Practise Yoga?'. Occasionally, the affirmation may stimulate a physical reaction within you, such as tears, shaking, heat, cold, shivers, embarrassment or fear. This is only the body releasing things that you have held within you from some time in your life when the only appropriate action seemed to be to shut your true feelings away. Hidden pain such as this may make you reluctant to use that affirmation, or indeed any affirmation, or make you feel foolish to say it. This shows that it is exactly the affirmation that you needed!—and that it is already working, in a deep way.

There is no need to get caught up in the reaction your body produces or to be concerned about it: just let it be there and remember White Eagle's words at the beginning of this chapter, 'Have you ever thought what forgiveness means…?', where he says that bitter and painful experiences grow more painful if you allow them to dominate you emotionally and mentally. The affirmation, when it brings such a reaction, is just working in a very deep way to release the held-in effect of these bitter and painful experiences, so that we no longer need to hold onto the memory of them or any resentments or fears about them. Again, it enables us to come truly into living in the here and now. For these fears and memories are held in the physical body in tension and tightness in the muscles and elsewhere, and can so easily be released through the physical body by the combining of yoga and affirmations, without our having to get caught up in the psychology of it all. It is not necessary even to know consciously what it is all about, much less to have to analyze and work it all out at an intellectual level. Just let the reaction be there; it will quickly pass as we continue with the affirmation, and there will be a feeling of lightness, relief and release, as a result.

So know within your heart that all is working within you to enable you to let go of what you have outgrown and no longer need. Just have faith and trust in this process of healing, and know that transformation *is* taking place and is guided by your own Higher Self. For as White Eagle tells us, we are only given at any one time what is within our own capacity to deal with.

It is often helpful to write down the affirmation, and next to it the feeling it gives you, and go on writing it day by day until there is no longer a reaction within you. You will then know that you really have been released from it. Just work on two or three affirmations at a time, otherwise there will be confusion.

Yama 1: Ahimsa (non-violence)

We see the human mind largely dominated by fear of the future, fear of the unknown. Surely you know by now that whatever tangle you find yourself in, whatever emotional strain is yours, these cannot last for ever, but are passing phases which come only as lessons to teach you something of value? You are here that you may learn, may gain knowledge which is essential to your well-being; and it is the actual experience of living with your fellow man which brings you wisdom.

Wisdom also comes direct from heaven as the result of your reaching upward to heaven, to higher planes of heavenly understanding; and wisdom says that bitter and painful experiences grow yet more painful if you allow them to disturb you emotionally and mentally. The alternative is to learn to lay them aside, and in everything to depend upon the love of God.

Confusion will depart if you can contact the Divine Heart by simple prayer uttered in faith and trust, and most of all in humility.

White Eagle, GOLDEN HARVEST

Ahimsa is most closely translated as 'non-violence', which implies not to kill, not to be angry, to control the violent, aggressive side of our natures; yet the wider, broader meaning of the word *ahimsa* is love embracing all, seeing ourselves and our fellow men and all creation as part of the whole, part of us—so loving all, that the destruction of any part of the earth or creation is the destruction of ourselves. So 'non-violence' encompasses seeing through all things with love, creating and affirming peace everywhere, knowing that that which manifests as violence only comes out of fear. If we can see through the fear and just *love*—whoever, wherever, whatever—then we in our hearts are practising *ahimsa*—non-violence.

We may look at the word 'non-violence' and say 'yes, I believe in non-violence' and then look at the world around us and say 'how terrible is the violence that manifests there—what on earth can we do about it?' Mahatma Gandhi, the world's greatest exponent of non-violence, said 'Look to yourselves, to the violence which manifests within yourself'. This may be a shock, to feel that we may have feelings of anger or violence hidden within us, yet look at the little ways it can come out unexpectedly in each one of us: in an angry word, or in uncontrollably lashing out at someone or something in our lives when we are caught off guard. For example, it is very easy to get frustrated and annoyed with other drivers on busy roads; at work when we feel misunderstood or put upon it is easy to see the other person as being in the wrong; or in the home when we are weary and feel we do not have the help we need we become resentful towards those close to us. Afterwards we feel guilty and sorry, but we do it again and again and often feel quite powerless to change.

Yet we could be helped to recognize and own these feelings if we accepted that they are partly a result of the frustrations of living on the earth in a very fast, over-sophisticated, over-busy society, confined to a limited physical body after being a free-flowing spirit. Somewhere within all of us there is the cry of a tiny, helpless baby waking up to the new conditions of separate earth life.

As we grow, all the restrictions that are put upon us as a little child (particularly when parents overdo this by modelling their own fears) reinforce the feelings held within us. Then in our adulthood these same fears and restrictions cause similar circumstances to reproduce themselves around us. Our Higher Self, we might say, is recreating these conditions in order for us to recognize the thought-patterns which we are holding onto and so release them. As White Eagle says, our outer circumstances are just what we need to grow strong in our spirit within and for it to shine through to the outer self.

This is where the practice of the last six limbs of yoga—the postures, the breathing, the control of the senses, and the three stages of meditation—have such a remarkable effect on our whole system. They work continuously to release the tension, fear and frustration that is held within us, so enabling us to practise the first two limbs of yoga—the *yamas* and the *niyamas*. The postures, particularly the dynamic ones such as the Warrior and Hero poses, have the power to dissolve the tension that since early childhood we have held onto in the muscles, the ligaments, and even the bones and organs of the body, thereby enabling us to bring out the positive attributes of the warrior and the hero, such as strength, courage, and dynamism, and to let go of the negative ones such as aggression and fear. Others that are particularly dynamic are all the rest of the standing poses, the back bends and the inverted poses.

With all forms of natural healing, the symptoms sometimes seem initially to get worse under treatment, seem to be more negative, or grow into nausea and shakiness. Although this can be quite upsetting, it is only the effect of the body, through the muscles, releasing the held-in hurts. Just let them surface and let them go, and continue practising the postures, and those feelings will quickly and progressively pass. Go on releasing them, for soon the body will feel much lighter and freer.

The breathing, *pranayama*, purifies and cleanses the blood, and clears the nervous system of fear and anxiety, both of which can create anger. Meditation enables us to feel at peace with ourselves and with the world and to be aware of the love within and around us.

Pratyahara, the control of the senses, enables us to detach ourselves from sudden, uncontrolled negative reactions to situations, and to be able to look at the situation in the true light of the spirit.

It is possible to practise the postures in a very physical way, straining with force and ambition to get into them—indeed yoga is sometimes taught in this way. If so, we lose the inner effect of the postures (such as those I have described for each one) and do not allow the energy to flow within the body as it moves through the postures. We then still hold much within us, building up a defence of tight muscles around us. So we need to remember that the postures have a much deeper effect than merely producing a strong, healthy, supple body, and to allow that effect to manifest.

Sometimes other techniques of personal release can be a great help when they are used in conjunction with the discipline of yoga: such therapies as the various forms of counselling, massage, bioenergetics, rebirthing, Gestalt therapies, acupuncture and shiatsu. I myself found the courses run by Universal Training (then the Self-Transformation Centre), in which many of these therapies are brought together, a great help in releasing a lot from the past. They also deepened my understanding of yoga and enabled me to see new ways in which it can help us in the West.

When we look deeply into the concept of non-violence we can understand that it actually means world peace—a state to which all those of us who would like to change the world are aspiring. There seem to me to be two ways of working for world peace. One is to visualize and affirm and creatively project it. In the White Eagle Lodge we use the powerful symbol of the six-pointed star, holding all difficult, unresolved situations in the world in the healing light of the Christ Star. Such a visualization has a very powerful effect on these situations and the politicians involved. At the other end of the spectrum are the very socially and politically activated people who want to do something practical: to send money, food, or clothing, or go into the situation for themselves and try to bring about change. Great beauty can come to the soul through so doing. Sometimes, however, there is aggression even in this. The most effective agent for peace is one who has looked at, understood and released aggressive feelings entirely. As a basis for either way of helping, the individual has the opportunity to recognize a very personal responsibility—his or her share in the collective consciousness that accommodates poverty, violence and pollution, thus perpetuating the suffering in our world and permitting the spoliation of it. In other words, we are all responsible for the whole.

If we look where our own fear and lack of trust come from and work on releasing them, as already described, we can be a much more powerful and effective instrument in sending out the light and also in helping at the practical level. Once each one of us can do this for ourselves in whatever way works for us, the world will be full of peace. An affirmation that would help is:

I let go of all anger; I release all resentment.
I see only peace; I am peace; I am divine peace.
I forgive myself, I forgive others (you can use names here); I see only love.

A beautiful affirmation, taken from LIVING IN THE LIGHT, by Shakti Gawain, is:

I am willing to learn to trust and follow my own inner truth, knowing that as I do, I will release the pain and fear within me and thus heal the pain and fear in the world.

Yama 2: Satya (truth)

Be true. This is the essence of the spiritual life. The note of your spirit is sounded on the higher planes, and the knocks you receive in everyday life are to test you, whether you can ring true. To ring true you must always sound the note of God, or good, which is within you.

White Eagle, THE QUIET MIND

Satya means 'truth'. The Sanskrit means much more than just not telling lies, to which it is often limited. Mahatma Gandhi said 'Truth is God, God is truth'. If we live in God we cannot help but be truthful. Being truthful in the yogic concept includes not ridiculing what others hold to be sacred, not telling tales, being true to our own Higher Self, having integrity with regard to our actions and interactions with others, having the courage to be open and authentic. The word 'integrity' seems to me to exemplify the much broader meaning of the word *satya*. 'Integrity', like 'honesty', also implies consistency: in integrity, there is nothing in what you say that contradicts what you think or do; no thought opposes any other thought, no act belies your word, and no word lacks agreement with any other. If we are whole and integrated within ourselves then we *are* truth.

An affirmation on truth:

I now have courage to see the truth in all.
I see from the light of the true self, the God-self within.

I feel safe in God's love.

Again, as in *ahimsa*, we need to look within ourselves to see if we are being true to the light within us, true to our own Inner Self. There are occasions in our interaction with others when we either impulsively or as a calculated 'cover-up' feel the need not to show our true selves, often for fear of what others may think or say about us, or because we judge them untrustworthy. At other times, we may find ourselves unable to be truthful to ourselves about our feelings, or ideas; or we may feel too much under the influence of other people's, or society's, opinions. Such thought-patterns may stem from a sense of inadequacy or guilt. Guilt causes us to cover up our true self for fear of being judged, by God, by others, and for fear of being judged, we judge ourselves. Yet, as White Eagle says, 'To ring true you must always sound the note of God, or good, which is within you'.

Looking into our hearts, we can see the light of the true self shining there clear and bright; and at the same time, we can recognize what prevents us from touching the true self. If we can see the obstacles just as collected dross that can be burnt away by the Higher Self, the candle flame within, then we can release all that prevents us from being constantly in touch with that self, the self that is pure and innocent.

The first of the *niyamas, saucha*, is a useful reference to this.

Yama 3: Asteya (non-stealing)

Giving means extending one's Love with no conditions, no expectations and no boundaries.
  Peace of mind occurs, therefore, when we put all our attention into giving and have no desire to get anything from, or to change, another person.
  The giving motivation leads to a sense of inner peace and joy that is unrelated to time.

Gerald Jampolsky, LOVE IS LETTING GO OF FEAR

As well as not taking that which belongs to others, *asteya* means not desiring to possess what another has, not envying others for their position, their fortune, their state of being. Again the theft which manifests in our society is something over which we ourselves have a responsibility. We draw such things to us by our fear, possessiveness and greed, which we all have in some measure. If we can feel content (a *niyama*) with ourselves, knowing that what we have is exactly what we need for our chosen path, we will not need to be envious of others or desirous for more. We can have what we need by being in touch with our source, our Higher Self; in this awareness, we can totally accept what we *do* have—which is not the same as being resigned to what we have. There needs to be a balance point between attaining and accepting.

Attainment, as soul-development, actually involves acceptance of where we are at any one time.

In the words of the familiar prayer:

God grant me the courage to change the things I can change; the serenity to accept those I cannot change; and the wisdom to know the difference.

If we turn *asteya*, non-stealing, around, we have giving—giving of our own free will and accord. Our society encourages us to take, to want more, to want something for nothing, to acquire possessions, certificates, degrees, bigger cars, better houses. This mental pattern encourages stealing as a manifestation of the distortion of society's views. If we could change our attitude to one of giving, believing that there is an abundant flow of life that comes from God through us in whatever form—be it love, money, possessions, time, understanding—then we would be released from the 'possessiveness' that manifests in our society.

Here is an affirmation:

All the abundance of the universe flows through me.
All my needs are abundantly fulfilled.

Yama 4: Brahmacharya (reverence for the creative life-force within)

Only in relationship can you know yourself, not in abstraction and certainly not in isolation.
The movement of behaviour is the sure guide to yourself, it's the mirror of your consciousness; this mirror will reveal its content, the images, the attachments, the fears, the loneliness, the joy and sorrow.
Poverty lies in running away from this, either in its sublimations or its identities.

KRISHNAMURTI'S JOURNAL

The dictionary translation of *brahmacharya* is 'celibacy'. To use this single western word with all its overtones is, I feel, to restrict this particular *yama* to the asceticism of only a few followers of yoga. B. K. S. Iyengar interprets the *brahmachari* (the yogi who practises *brahmacharya*) as a person who constantly has his or her being in God, and knows that all exists in God, and so is aware of the divinity in all living beings and in the whole earth.

Both White Eagle and Mr Iyengar say that without experiencing human love and happiness, it is not possible to know divine love. Here are some other quotations that may illuminate this *yama*:

Human love
is not a substitute for spiritual love.
It is an extension of it.

Each lifetime
and each relationship within each lifetime
is an opportunity to experience love.

When you see each other
as the Divine and eternal beings that you are,
you will never cease to wonder and to glory
in the coming together. Do not be seduced
into seeing each other merely as the human shell.
Rather, see the soul, the consciousness within.

EMMANUEL'S BOOK

If you would learn the secret of right relations, look only for the good, that is, the divine, in people and things, and leave all the rest to God.

J. Allen Boone, KINSHIP WITH ALL LIFE

Many of the ancient mystery schools as well as modern-day Buddhist and Christian monasteries and other religious schools require the aspirant to be celibate, yet I feel that only for a few devotees is this the natural state of being, and that it does not need to be imposed upon people who are unwilling; for when it is forced and the feeling nature is repressed many problems are created. In our current state of evolution there is generally a need for us to deal with the feeling side of our natures and to learn to live in harmony with it, in ourselves and in others.

All the teachers that I have quoted emphasize that being in relationship with others is an integral part of our earth-experience and of our being on a spiritual path, but stress that we need to enter partnership with great reverence for the creative life-force that is within each one of us.

As a society we have divorced our sexuality from God, we have tended to treat sex just as a sensation to be experienced on the physical level. To clarify Krishnamurti's words, we identify with the sensation it gives us on a feeling level, and get caught up in an apparent desire and need for that sensation. At the other extreme, sexuality and sensuality get regarded as base, unclean, a weakness to which we see ourselves or others giving way, one which we tend to condemn, and so attempt to sublimate or repress in various ways.

On the path of yoga or any spiritual path many aspirants, myself included, have found it beneficial for some time to practise celibacy in order to become aware of the true nature of the divine life-force within and so develop a true reverence and respect for the creative life-principle. A time of self-control and self-assessment can certainly be helpful, particularly as yoga can be and has been misused in such a way as to stir up the powerful creative life-force, to the point of its being out of control. That this should happen is often an indication that it was repressed in the first place. So long as the self-control comes out of respect and reverence for this deep creative life-force rather than as a repression of the life-force at a feeling level, there will be no difficulties in asserting self-control; but repression always leads either to sudden uncontrolled outbursts or to problems within the physical body, psyche and emotional body.

The old, old question of self-control as against creative self-expression is one that current generations are very much working on. It seems to me as though many of us, particularly those who grew up in the revolution of the Sixties which rejected enforced discipline and broke down the strict Victorian codes of morality, needed to discover through our own experience the exact nature of our feelings and our sexuality and for a time explore them, in order to find the true nature of this deep creative life-force within us. A great reassessment has gone on since those days. It is very evident from the media that the trend-setters of that time in the pop and fashion world now follow a vastly different lifestyle, many of them choosing celibacy for a time and advocating a deep reverence for the creative life-principle. If we all regarded our sexuality as the highest creative force within us, giving us the potential for complete at-one-ment with another being, and therefore ultimately with God, we would not have the need to restrain or repress ourselves, neither would there be all the misuse of sex seen in our society.

White Eagle says:

Do not be in too much of a hurry, dear children, to rush on and find the next thrill. The desire body is powerful and it desires fresh excitements. The disciple on the path moves forward slowly.

This desire to rush on can apply to all aspects of life, physical and spiritual—perhaps we need to slow down and examine more closely what we think we need and desire, to see if this is our hearts' true want and need, or just a current sensation on the feeling level. We may also then see what is blocking us from having what we desire—it may well be just our own thought-patterning. Every spiritual teacher that I know of says that we only need trust in God, trust in our Higher Selves, to know our greatest good, and all we ever need or want will come to us. It is, I feel, through this trust and faith in God that 'desirelessness' comes, because if we trust that all we want or need will come to us when the time is right, then we have no need to yearn for our desires to be met.

The practice of the postures of yoga can work towards this

detachment from desires, but it is all still *our* choice—in the way that we work and what we do with this creative energy. Yet it is possible to transcend what we think of as base desires, created at the feeling level, and take them to a much higher level of pure love from the heart. Then there is no misuse of this very precious creative energy. So if in the postures and the breathing we concentrate on drawing the life-force up from the basal centres to the heart centre, the more the desires produced in these centres are no longer repressed but transcended and we communicate in love, from the heart.

Indian art in temples and sacred sites is a combination of the religious and the mystical, with the sensual and the erotic. This often makes the Westerner and the westernised Indian very uncomfortable: we see these aspects as completely separate because our energy centres are not integrated. We cut ourselves off from our body and its sensations; we are mostly centred in our heads.

The subconscious is said to reside in the pelvic region, in the basal and sacral centres.* We tend to push it down there if we find it unacceptable to the conscious mind, the mind in the head. However, it tends to come out in unpredictable ways, in our dreams, in our meditation and contemplation, in thoughts which can shock and disturb the conscious mind, in unexpected reactions to people or events which touch on our subconscious. These buried feelings also come out in our society as, for example, debauchery, rape or pornography.

The practice of the postures, by allowing the energy to rise gradually from the base centres upwards in a safe, gentle way, integrates the subconscious mind with the conscious mind. This integration allows both to let go their hold of us so that henceforth we are centred in the mind in the heart—the meeting-place and blending of the conscious and subconscious.

So there comes to be an understanding and at-one-ment with the body and its innate intelligence. This helps us to be in touch with the real creative source within us and so be true to it. We will then not require sex as a sensation but as a true act of union or love. So also there is discipline, without suppression of our feeling nature, but which stems from always being true to our Inner Self. We may also find that through true self-understanding we become naturally celibate because we have transcended sexual energies. This can be recognized in some of the spiritual teachers, who emanate pure love from the heart with no repression of their feeling nature. It can also be reflected in a monogamous relationship which acknowledges that desire can exist outside that relationship, without the need to follow that desire.

A helpful affirmation would be something like:

I trust in the creative process of life, I see love everywhere and in everyone.
I feel free to express the joy of life.
I let go of my desires and trust that all I ever need or want will come to me.

Do create your own affirmations for your own circumstances, for they are far more effective and powerful if they touch on what you need to lead you into a joyous realization of this divine love in every aspect of your life.

*For further comments about this, see Joan Hodgson's *The Stars and the Chakras*

Yama 5: Aparigraha (non-possessiveness)

Personal love of a selfless nature is beautiful and it makes life lovely and brings great happiness. But the personal love must be broad and wide. Love, like power, must be poised; it must be steady; it must in a sense be impersonal. You may think that impersonal love is cold, but this is not so. Impersonal love is pure and without condemnation; it is all-embracing, all-enfolding, all-tenderness. Above all, it is love without pain....

Love thy neighbour, love thy God. All selfish desire, all desire to have and to hold must go; you must be prepared to lose, to give—all. This does not mean that all will of necessity be demanded of you, but rather that desire for possession must fall away.

White Eagle, GOLDEN HARVEST

Aparigraha means 'non-possessiveness', non-hoarding. One of the effects of fear is that we regard those whom we love, together with our material goods, as something we could lose, and we cling to them. True unconditional love is not possessive either of people or objects, but love without thought of what we get in return. True love of the heart does not say 'I will love if....': it accepts and loves without condition: this is non-possessiveness. This means to love under all circumstances, even when we feel threatened or fearful, which is not always easy: yet if we can see through our own immediate reaction when hurt or disturbed and feel from our hearts the love that is there both within ourselves and within others we can let go of the hurt. Initially, this can involve a great effort, yet as soon as we touch that infinite well of love in the heart all else becomes insignificant.

Non-hoarding is not collecting clutter around us, for that clutter in the outer world is representative of the clutter in our outer minds that prevents us from touching the true spirit within. There is a book by Don Aslett called FREEDOM FROM CLUTTER that recommends that we throw away anything that we have not used for two years. I find this a good policy in daily life. How good it feels to clear out a cupboard, to throw away all that we do not need, use or love, because when we do this we are indeed 'clearing ourselves out' inside! That is why it feels so refreshing, relieving: it is symbolic of clearing out the dark cluttered corners of ourselves. The postures and the breathing of yoga, too, have this cleansing, clearing effect in the body, an effect which makes space, lightness and openness around us.

For this reason many yogis of the East do not have a permanent residence: they carry all they need on their backs. Hoarding comes out of fear, and if we let go of fear then we can trust that our every need will be provided for by God, by the universe, in both our outer and Inner Selves.

Insecurity begins when the little child discovers it is not still in the womb and suddenly feels separate from its mother, separate from the universe. As long as the mother is there to hold and comfort the tiny babe, the child gradually becomes secure again and feels safe in the world. But many of the theories about bringing up children—now mostly discarded—such as leaving a baby in a cot to cry, have reinforced such insecurities in us. We suffer from such a degree of insecurity that we clutter ourselves with insurances, pensions, mortgages, fences, walls, defence systems. This insecurity is locked into the sacrum bone, the sacral centre (see the section on the chakras and centres) in our bodies. Movements in the hip area in the postures free this sacred sacrum bone gradually so that we can let go of these insecurities and fears. Such postures as the Triangle and the Stretched Flank, the Cobbler, *janu sirsasana* and others, free the sacrum bone very gently, and have the effect of turning us inward to a trust in our Higher Selves, in God and the universe for our security and safe-keeping; breathing in the creative life-force that sustains us.

If we can touch and feel that oneness of all life, and know that we are a child of the universe, one with the universe, we release all insecurities. This comes through meditation on the oneness, or unity, of all life.

Aparigraha encompasses not taking what one does not really need, nor taking things without working for them—this indicates poverty of spirit. Favours given and taken can often come out of a desire to possess someone or something.

God provides all our needs when we remain in touch with our Source and do all we need for ourselves, and let go of desires. An affirmation is helpful, such as:

I let go of all fears, I trust in the process of my life.
I put my trust in God to provide all my needs.
I open to life, I love life.'

II. *Niyamas*

Following the five *yamas*—living with regard for others and to our Highest Self—are the *niyamas*.

The *niyamas* are concerned with how we live our life with regard to ourselves, caring for and loving ourselves. We do not find it easy to love ourselves, but how can we love others if we do not love and accept ourselves as we are, at the same time looking at and working on our own growth and development? Again an affirmation is helpful, such as:

I love and accept myself as I am, as a divine, perfect being full of God's love.

Niyama 1: Saucha (purity)

*I will forgive all things today, that I
May learn how to accept the truth in me,
And come to recognize my sinlessness.*

A COURSE IN MIRACLES, lesson 119

The perfect man, the master soul, is a very wonderful and glorious being. You are that being, in embryo....

All life consists of two aspects, which can be variously called positive and negative, constructive and destructive, light and darkness, good and evil.... Your heart, which is your true self, longs for and believes in truth, believes in a heaven world, and in God's goodness; it accepts these as a little child does, feeling and knowing that they are true. Another part of you is of the earth, and pulls you down again, so that what you may believe in tonight, tomorrow you cannot spare time for.... You, the real you, are here for a purpose, to shine through both body and mind and transmute them.... Your own body, seen with the eye of the spirit, is a form composed of clear light.

Many will presently be helped to realize this by science, which has now concluded that not only is there no solidity in matter—truth which was known long, long ago by the Wise Men—but has almost determined that physical matter does not really exist, that it is what the Easterners call 'maya' or illusion. We are told, however, that when the physical atom, with its electrons and protons, is examined by the eye of the spirit, it is seen that around the protons are particles of light. Thus within the physical atom the light shines, and without that light there would be no atom and no world in which form could exist.

White Eagle, MORNING LIGHT

Saucha means 'purity'. A very powerful and evocative word; for we are of spirit, and therefore pure, innocent and divine in mind, body and spirit. Yet there is the darker side to acknowledge so that it may in due course become bathed in light.

The philosophy of yoga teaches that at any one moment we are perfect—whole and complete; and yet we are on the karmic wheel, likened in eastern philosophy to the symbol for infinity, ∞, or a figure 8. At whatever point we are on that wheel all is just as it should be and just as it needs to be at that moment, in whatever conditions we find ourselves and whatever the state of our minds and bodies. What White Eagle says is that the conditions of our life at any one moment are exactly what we need for us to evolve and grow. All we need to do is accept the conditions of our lives at the precise moment in which we experience them, most especially to accept our own self in all its aspects; through this acceptance we are able to overcome our inner and outer difficulties without the need for stress or strain. This is absolutely analogous to our practice of yoga in whatever form that is expressed.

Western theologians have given us a very different viewpoint; in their teaching (to a greater or lesser extent) we are born in sin, we are all sinners and we therefore need to strive for repentance. Actually, at the root of the word repentance, beyond even its Latin derivation, is the sense 'return to the source'—return to God. It means to look again to our God-self, our Inner Self, our Higher Self. A totally different meaning from the one we have put on it.

As White Eagle says in the quotation, it is the earth, or these earth-bound beliefs, that create the feeling of being a sinner, and perhaps what we call the darker side of our nature; this is our outer mind—not the body which has a natural intelligence and purity of its own. Were not we made in the image of God?

Be ye therefore perfect, even as your Father which is in heaven is perfect.

Matthew 5: 48

The postures and the breathing of yoga help to cleanse negative thoughts and beliefs from our system, so clearing out toxins, cleansing the blood and nervous system. The toxins accumulate from held-in negative beliefs and fears, and once we release them our whole system becomes pure and clear. So we no longer want to eat foods that clog up our system. A strongly-imprinted belief of impurity may manifest as a need to eat heavy foods, such as meat, sugar, refined and preserved foods, and consume stimulating drinks, drugs and tobacco, to reinforce this held-in belief, which is why many strict diets do not work and there is a great tendency to go back to old habits as soon as we come off the diet. These old habits may run through families and generations. What is advocated by dietary experts at any one time changes. Often what is the current advice has its root in the collective beliefs of that time, and as those beliefs change our eating habits change.

The only way we can really change our eating habits and our living habits is to change ourselves and release any negative beliefs and cramping emotions held deep within us. To release the negativity we need to own it, accept it, embrace it and love it. Giving ourselves time each day to do our yoga and meditation practice can be part of caring for, accepting and loving ourselves. This is not selfish, a criticism often levelled at spiritual practices such as yoga, because giving ourselves this time greatly helps us to live in the world with others. Through the practice of yoga we naturally want to eat pure, healthy fresh food: sunshine-filled food, fruits, vegetables, nuts, pulses, clear spring water. However, it is not necessary to force our systems in any way, we need to eat that which makes us salivate, that which really tastes good to us, noting if it makes us feel good. If a particular food does not make you feel good, then next time you feel inclined to eat it, pause and ask your body if it really wants it, if it would really appreciate the food and be nurtured by it. Tune in to your body's responses—if your body is telling you that it would not be good for you, by recurrent tuning in you will begin actually not to want the food that is of no value to you.

Try saying to yourself:

I am pure, I am innocent, I am divine.

This may bring up a lot of feelings of lack of these qualities. By not attaching yourself to them you just let them pass by. Watch them go: and so cleanse your whole self.

Niyama 2: Santosa (contentment)

To trust God means that you are absolutely at peace. You see life as a process of growth, and what appears so ugly and distressing you see as a condition which will ultimately bring beauty and perfection in the life of man.

If you have confidence in God you will remain untouched by anything the world can do. You will no longer be confused and troubled, once you have found confidence in God.

Nothing is real except the love and wisdom of God. You say, 'But the problem of suffering is very real to those who are passing through it!'. But we answer, the one who is suffering can find relief from that suffering through complete surrender to the goodness and love of God. Suffering comes because the individual is unaware of the presence of God; he is separate, alienated from the love of God....

Try to realize that Christ's kingdom is in you, and also that you live in it, in Christ's kingdom of the Star. If you can realize this perfect life within, in time it must manifest in your life, in your surroundings. This is the natural law ... as above, so below; as below, so above.

White Eagle, THE GENTLE BROTHER

Santosa is a beautiful word, meaning 'contentment': acceptance of where we are in life, which is exactly where we need to be for our evolution. Deep inner contentment comes from having faith in God, faith in our own Higher Self, faith in the process of life. It is inner knowledge that our Higher Self has chosen to be where it is to learn, to work through our karma, to live our life, to fulfil our potential. If we live true to our Selves and trust in God, all will come to us, every need will be met, every desire of the heart fulfilled. We do not need to be 'in need', we choose to *be*.

The practice of yoga, the study of ancient teaching such as White Eagle's, and the meditation that is common to both, gradually give this deep inner contentment and choice to be as we are and where we are. An affirmation that would be helpful at the end of meditation, if this concept is not easy for you, is:

I am content in myself, in God.
I accept my life as it is and live it to the full potential of my Higher Self, my God Self.

Niyama 3: Tapas (being alive with enthusiasm)

When you are inspired by some great purpose, some extraordinary project, all your thoughts break their bonds; your mind transcends limitations, your consciousness expands in every direction, and you find yourself in a new, great and wonderful world. Dormant forces, faculties and talents become alive, and you discover yourself to be a greater person by far than you ever dreamed yourself to be.

Yoga commentary, quoted in Susan Hayward, A GUIDE FOR THE ADVANCED SOUL

The Sanskrit root of *tapas* means 'to blaze'. This is the inner fire that urges us on to develop, to achieve, to love life and all that we do. For example, if we have not got our heart in the practice of yoga, if it is just (say) a weekly class of stretching and relaxation because it makes us feel better or we feel we ought to do it, then it will not do much for us. There needs to be a great inner desire to practise yoga, to achieve oneness, unity with all. Without that inner fire we may as well forget it.

There are many apparent reasons why people first attend a yoga class or buy a book on yoga—apparent reasons, because we are not always in touch with that inner fire that urges us on. Yet the inner fire is there and directs our life in subtle ways, ways of which we are not always aware. For instance we might go to a class because of a bad back, headaches, or feelings of stress and tension. Yoga works on all of these but the outer manifestations and troubles are often the body urging us to do something to change something in our lives; to free ourselves from the hold the outer body has on us. If we abuse our body, it will rebel. Disease is our body letting us know that it has had enough and that something needs to change. So initially yoga works to bring to the surface the problem, the pain, the dis-ease, and truly anything is possible with yoga (see 'Good and Bad Pain', p. 56). Through this we become aware of the desire to change, release, develop. Once we are in touch with that inner desire, *tapas*, it no longer becomes an effort, something we have to force ourselves to do—we really want to do it, from a deep, inner knowing of its true effect and true meaning. This takes us onto the next *niyama*. A helpful affirmation would be:

I touch the source of the divine fire in me and let it work in my life.

Niyama 4: Svadhyaya (self-study)

The way to truth is through the spirit. In the outer world there is turmoil and chaos and unhappiness. You think with the mortal mind, with the mind which is part of the substance of earth. You should think with your inner mind, you should approach problems through the inner self, through intuition. The very word explains itself. In-tuition— training inside yourself. You are looking outside for help, and all the time the help you want is inside. The world of spirit that so many of you talk about and believe in, and long to touch, is all within.

White Eagle, THE QUIET MIND

The Self is all-knowing,
    it is all-understanding,
      and to it belongs all glory.
It is pure consciousness,
    dwelling in the heart of all,
      in the divine citadel of Brahma.
There is no space it does not fill.

Dwelling deep within,
    it manifests as mind,
      silently directing the body and the senses.
The wise behold this Self,
    blissful and immortal,
      shining forth through everything.

MUNDAKA UPANISHAD

The Upanishad here refers to the Self with a capital 'S', meaning the divine spark of God within, also referred to as the Higher or Inner Self.

Svadhyaya is 'self-study', not in the sense of absorption in the little self but in the sense of touching that source of knowledge that is within. Yoga works on the precept that all the knowledge in the universe is within us, it just needs bringing out; we just have to remember what we have always known. This is totally opposite to the orthodox Western education system, that teaches and imprints knowledge into us from a specific, rigid frame of reference built up over just a few hundred years. The knowledge that is within us is timeless, goes backwards and forwards over all time and taps into all sources. White Eagle calls this knowledge the Ancient Wisdom, which is the source of all spiritual teaching and runs through all religions. It is evident in Egypt, in Atlantis, in the Tao, in yoga, in esoteric Christianity, and elsewhere. It is the basis for the complete understanding of our evolution on all levels. We just need to go within and ask in humility to be shown the way. That is not to say that we do not need a teacher in yoga,

especially in the first years of practice, and yet as Richard Bach says, teaching is only reminding people what they already know. However, a teacher who works from the heart can help us break through the belief of the outer mind that there is a 'right' and a 'wrong' way, a 'correct' or 'incorrect' way, and so help us touch our source of knowledge, of intuition.

It is interesting to separate the word intuition as White Eagle does: in-tuition, or tuition from within. So yoga develops the intuition, the capacity to know exactly what our body and soul need at any one time. But we can also see others clearly by means of intuition: know their needs, their difficulties, their dis-ease, and be able to help. The awareness required in teaching yoga is developed by the aspiring teacher's practice on himself or herself, which taps into his or her inner knowing. When constantly in tune with his or her intuition a teacher can always find a way to help by picking up intuitively from his or her own practice what is needed in each pupil. This not only applies in the practice of yoga, but also in life itself—for yoga is analagous to life—and what is right for one person is not necessarily right for another.

Acceptance of this precept teaches us tolerance towards all, however unacceptable another's behaviour may seem, outwardly.

So as long as the teacher has been true in his or her own practice, he or she can stand in front of a class and know the needs of the group, and be aware of specific individual needs. So *svadhyaya* is honestly, clearly looking at oneself—a yogi 'reads his own book of life, at the same time that he writes it and revises it'. These words are Mr Iyengar's, in LIGHT ON YOGA, although Mr Iyengar also recommends that we study divine literature in a pure place to help solve the problems of life.

Helpful affirmations would be:

I am divine knowledge.
All is within me.
All knowing is within me.

or

I trust my own inner knowing, my own intuition.

Niyama 5: Isvara Pranidhana (dedicating one's actions to God)

Great White Spirit of the open spaces, the mountain tops and the quiet peaceful valleys; Great White Spirit of nature and of the heavens above the earth, and of the waters beneath. Great White Spirit of eternity, infinity, we are enfolded within thy great heart. We rest our heart upon thy heart. Great Father and Mother God, we love, we worship thee; we resign all into thy loving keeping, knowing that thou art love, and all moves forward into the light.

White Eagle, PRAYER IN THE NEW AGE

Isvara is the Supreme Being, God. *Isvara pranidhana* means dedicating our actions, our development, to a higher source, a higher purpose. So all this practice is not done only for the earthly self, the lower self, but is dedicated to our view of a higher purpose, whether that be God, the upliftment of mankind, the planet as a whole, or in service to those around us. This idea of a higher source expands our whole vision to encompass not only those closest to us—not only our family and friends—but the whole earth, the universe itself; and brings this awareness of the oneness of all life. Such devotion to a higher Source is the essence of *bhakti* yoga—the yoga of devotion; in *bhakti*, B.K.S. Iyengar says, the mind, the intellect and the will are surrendered to the Lord. The practice of *bhakti* yoga is in the form of prayers, such as the beautiful prayer of White Eagle's above, a prayer which opens the heart to the Lord and surrenders all to the whole; and many people practise *bhakti* yoga without realizing it. In hymns, in music, and in songs to the divine, an organisation like the White Eagle Lodge practises *bhakti* yoga. Yet the postures, and other forms of yoga, encompass *bhakti* yoga too, if they are dedicated to God, and to the development of our Higher Self, called in yoga the *atman*.

Through yoga, the *atman* eventually becomes one with Brahman, Brahman being the highest aspect of God, unimaginable to the human mind.

Helpful affirmations here would be:

I commit all my actions to a higher purpose—to God.

I dedicate my life, my practice of yoga and all the deeds of my life to God.

The next six stages help us to achieve the first two stages, which are necessary precepts for the life of a yogi.

III. *Asanas* (postures)

Ancient wisdom teaches that the two forces of light and darkness both have an important part to play in the human soul. This idea will be familiar to students of yoga who gradually learn how to balance within themselves the lifestreams of the sun and the moon, the sun of course being positive or light, the moon negative or dark.

It is perhaps natural to associate light with goodness and darkness with evil, yet White Eagle's account of these two forces is rather different. He relates the sun lifestream to the outer life, to that part of us which is active and in control during the daylight or waking hours. The sun vitalises every part of our being, and more especially gives light and vitality to the physical body until the solar body, the body of light, can fully manifest through it.

The lunar lifestream or the dark self White Eagle relates to the invisible part of our being, which becomes more active during the hours of darkness when the conscious self is at rest; the subconscious and superconscious mind.

Joan Hodgson, PLANETARY HARMONIES

Yoga works on the principle that the body exactly reflects what is in the mind and in the emotions and buried in the subconscious. The body is a temple for the spirit, yet the outer body relates to the outer mind and to the emotions. So work on the body also works in the mind and emotions and removes blocks in these areas. In another of Mr Iyengar's books, THE TREE OF YOGA, we read:

> The science of yoga helps us to keep the body as a temple so that it becomes as clean as the soul. The body is lazy, the mind is vibrant and the soul is luminous. Yogic practices develop the body to the level of the vibrant mind so that the body and mind, having both become vibrant, are drawn towards the light of the soul.*

Philosophers, saints and sages tell us that there are various paths by which we can reach the ultimate goal, the sight of the soul. The science of mind is called *raja-yoga*, the science of intelligence is *jnana-yoga*, the science of duty is *karma-yoga*, and the science of will is *hatha-yoga*. For the authors of the ancient texts, these names were like the keys on a keyboard. The keyboard has many keys but the music is one. Similarly, there are many words by which individuals express their particular ways of approaching yoga and the particular paths through which they reach the culmination of their art, but yoga is one, just as God is one though in different countries people call Him by different names.

Those who approach yoga intellectually say that *raja-yoga* is spiritual and *hatha-yoga* merely physical. This is a tremendous misconception. As all paths lead towards the source, *hatha-yoga* too takes one towards the sight of the soul....

'Ha' means sun, which is the sun of your body, that is to say your soul, and 'tha' means moon, which is your consciousness. The energy of the sun never fades, whereas the moon fades every month and again from fading comes to fullness. So the sun in all of us, which is our soul, never fades, whereas the mind or consciousness, which draws its energy from the soul, has fluctuations, modulations, moods, ups and downs like the phases of the moon; it is like quicksilver, and as quicksilver

*In this passage, where Mr Iyengar uses the word 'soul' White Eagle readers will be more accustomed to the word 'spirit'.

cannot be caught by the hand, so we cannot easily catch hold of the mind. Yet when consciousness and the body are brought into union with one another, the energy of consciousnes becomes still and when the energy of consciousness is still, consciousness too is still, and the soul pervades the entire body.

In wanting to achieve the union that 'yoga' means it is tempting to feel that all we need is to touch the higher self, the *atman*, and we are there. But union means union on *all* levels, what White Eagle would call 'the spirit reigning supreme in the kingdom of the self'. This involves total self-acceptance, the whole being working as one in a union of the divine with the little self, as represented by the two triangles of the six-pointed star united and without division.

The postures have a very important part to play in this union, at a very subtle level; for they do have the effect of stirring up, and thus integrating what is held in the subconscious; as well as allowing us to recognize the source of our emotional reactions. The care and time spent on disciplining the physical body through the postures of yoga brings love and acceptance of the body—the temple of the spirit—that we have been given for our time on earth.

Posture of course includes the way we habitually stand, sit and hold ourselves. This makes such a difference to the way we feel. Shoulders hunched as though we are carrying a great load upon them, not trusting to God to hold it, are a symptom of collapse in the chest and heart areas, felt inwardly as depression. As soon as we train the body to lift and extend upwards in alignment and balance the depression lifts. On the other hand, if we stand very rigidly—sergeant-major stance—our mind and outlook will tend to be this way too, so that we are rigid and overbearing with others.

Through the postures we strengthen and straighten the spine, bringing a balance of strength and suppleness, establishing firmness on the earth at the same time as the whole body aspires to the heavens.

The branch of yoga that includes the postures is known as *hatha* yoga. *Hatha* means forcefully bringing one's will to bear on whatever we want to do. Although we can practise the postures in a forceful way and perhaps need at one time or another to break through the outer resistance of the body, there is a subtle balance to be found. It is interesting to split the word as Mr Iyengar does, into *Ha*, the sun, and *Tha*, the moon. To expand the interpretation already given by Mr Iyengar, we may add that *Ha* is traditionally associated with the masculine energies within us, and *Tha* with the feminine energies. In the practice of the postures we bring balance to these energies within us. The masculine energies (which both sexes possess) are those outgoing, dynamic 'doing' energies—the feminine energies are inward-turning, nurturing, quiet, 'being' energies. (There is more about these energies in chapter 2, the section on the chakras.)

Both are necessary in both male and female for balance. Some psychology states that the left side of the brain is the logical, rational, thinking side, and hence more masculine, and that it controls the right side of the body; the right side of the brain is the creative, intuitive, feeling side, and so more feminine, and it controls the left side of the body. These patterns can be reversed in some people. More recent research is showing that there is some interchange and that it is not as simple as previously suggested. In yoga, there is considered to be a subtle interchange of these energies up and down the spine, from right to left and left to right across the body. The movement in the postures moves and aligns and integrates these energies to give wholeness and balance. This would eventually merge the two halves of our brain into one complete whole, completely connected with our body.

I always remember Mr Iyengar saying in his classes, 'spread your intelligence to every cell of your body'. This is a strange concept for us when we are accustomed to believe that our intellect resides in our brains. Intelligence is much broader and wider than the intellect and can be there in every cell. If through the postures we bring aliveness and awareness to every cell then every cell will be intelligent. This is the purpose of the postures.

We live in a patriarchal society, and although this is changing very fast, it still demonstrates masculine energy in its forcefulness and strongly-held attitudes. Hence in most people the right side of the body leads, is stronger and more alive. We need to be aware of this in our practice of the postures and in daily life work to awaken the left side, our feminine energies. So sometimes a little more concentration on this side of the body is called for. It can be helpful to practise a posture to the left first, then to the right and then again to the left. At the second time of going to the left the body will be much more aware of the flow between the two sides. The practice of *hatha* yoga is the pathway to *raja* yoga, which, as its Sanskrit title indicates, is the king of the yogas; that is, attainment of union between the divine in ourselves and in the universe.

We can feel this union in the postures, which are rituals, prayers, supplications of the temple—the body that houses the spirit. The postures keep the temple of the body in perfect order: fit to house the spirit, at the same time as putting us in touch with that spirit by the deep concentration required in the postures.

IV. *Pranayama* (breathing)

One of the finest methods of which we knew in our American Indian days for the strengthening of the finer bodies and nervous system was by deep breathing. People little realise the importance of breathing correctly, and how the art of breathing can be used to cleanse and revivify not only the physical but every part of man's being.... As you breathe, realise that you are breathing not only air but the very life atoms into your being!....

You breathe in and absorb this stream of life and light from the Father-Mother God, and then you let it fall from you in blessing upon others. So you absorb God's life and you bless all life. You receive and you give; and so you come into harmony with the rhythmic lifestream. It will feed your nerves, and give you a sense of peace and control.

White Eagle, in SUN-MEN OF THE AMERICAS, by Grace Cooke

Pranayama, the third limb of yoga, means the extension and control of the breath. We tend to think of breathing as purely a mechanism of the lungs to take oxygen in and let carbon dioxide out of our body. Yet the breath is much more subtle than this— every cell of our body, every pore of our skin, breathes in this wonderful life-giving air, *prana*. When you concentrate on and think of the breath, when you can be *with* the breath, you can feel what a wonderful being you are and what an amazing and wonderful energy this life-giving force is.

In *pranayama* we concentrate on the breath, not to force it in any way but gradually to bring awareness of how to increase that life-giving energy. We can do this initially just by becoming aware of it, as explained in chapter 8, which is the practice section on relaxation and *pranayama*.

Pranayama helps and encourages the first two limbs—the *yamas* and the *niyamas*. Being aware of the breath puts us in touch with the divine spirit, the light within us. So if we find ourselves in a situation in which we feel uncomfortable or we are not reacting in the way we would like, if we just bring our awareness to our breathing, just touching that light within and going with our breath as it comes and goes, then the lack of ease will go, and we will become more in command of our reactions. Controlling the breath in *pranayama* gives a constant awareness of that divinity within us. To lead into and during *pranayama*, it is good to practise *asanas* to open the cells of the body and the chest area, to lengthen and straighten the spine, so that we can breathe fully.

Pranayama leads naturally into meditation, for which it is an excellent preparation. It is said that a yogi's life is not measured by years but by the number of breaths, and that this is why they live so long—the slow, rhythmic, steady breathing brought about by the daily practice of *pranayama* prolongs life and increases well-being.

V. *Pratyahara* (control of the senses)

Imagine the self as the rider in a chariot.
The body is the chariot,
*   the intellect the driver,*
*   and the mind the reins.*
The senses are the horses,
*   and their objects are the road.*
*   The Self, say the wise,*
when combined with the senses and the mind
*   becomes 'the enjoyer'.*

When a man lacks wisdom
*   his mind is always restless,*
*   and his senses are wild horses*
*   dragging the driver hither and thither.*

But when he is full of wisdom
*   his mind is collected,*
*   and his senses become tamed horses*
*   obedient to the driver's will....*

Subtler than the organs of perception are the senses.
Subtler than this is the mind.
Subtler than this is the intellect.
Subtler than this is the self.
Subtler than this is the underlying cause of all.

And subtler still is the supreme Self.
There is nothing subtler than this.
This is the Absolute.
This is the end of all suffering

The self lies hidden,
And is not openly displayed.
But It is known to those of subtle sight,
  whose vision is purified and clear.

The wise man's senses are governed by his mind.
His mind is governed by his intellect.
His intellect is governed by his active self.
And his active self is governed by the silent Self.

Wake up!
Seek the Truth!
Rise above ignorance!
Search out the best teachers,
  and through them find the Truth.
But beware!
  'The path is narrow', the sages warn
  'sharp as a razor's edge,
  most difficult to tread'.

KATHA UPANISHAD, Part 3

The Upanishads are *sutras* on yoga, the earliest dating from around 800 B.C., written by the then forest dwellers of India.

In the context of the present book, let us substitute 'the intelligence' for 'the intellect' in this passage.

Pratyahara means 'control of the senses'. We have a tendency always to be looking for new and different sensations, be they food, drink, drugs, fast cars, sex, new experiences; but are these sensations deeply satisfying or just for the passing moment? *Pratyahara* means looking at those sensations to see if we really want them, if they are really going to be of benefit to us.

This aspect comes under *kriya* yoga, the practice of complete withdrawal from the world of the senses; an inward turning, away from the feeling body; a refusal to be at its beck and call. This, for us in the western world, is rather extreme, but we can still practise *pratyahara* in gentler ways by looking at the habits we have in life that do not make us feel good; that make us declare 'I wish I hadn't done that', that are not beneficial to our whole selves. These habits are not only the extreme ones of diet, drug-dependence, or irresponsible sexual activity, but things such as wallowing in emotion and drama. If we note these tendencies in ourselves, just observe them, it is very helpful to write down the feelings we have about them. Then the next time we feel the urge to indulge, we can bring to the mind the aftermath, the feelings that follow, and so be much less inclined to indulge in excesses.

It is better not to be too forceful, too extreme about this, but to be very patient, as one would when training a highly sensitive horse. Often observation of ourselves over a period of time is enough for the habit to go gently and easily. If you lapse, do not be too severe, because anything that is merely suppressed will break out again. However, we can change when we really want to, and the postures, the breathing and meditation bring this about gradually and without strain or force in all areas of our life.

The Three Stages of Meditation

Meditation is not for him who eats too much, nor for him who eats not at all: nor for him who is overmuch addicted to sleep, nor for him who is always awake.

But for him who regulates his food and recreation, who is balanced in action, in sleeping and in waking, it shall dispel all unhappiness.

When the mind, completely controlled, is centred in the Self, and free from all earthly desires, then is the man truly spiritual.

The wise man who has conquered his mind and is absorbed in the Self is as a lamp which does not flicker, since it stands sheltered from every wind.

There, where the whole nature is seen in the light of the Self, where the man abides within his self and is satisfied, there, its functions restrained by its union with the Divine, the mind finds rest.

BHAGAVAD GITA, chapter VI

The Bhagavad Gita, an ancient Hindu text and part of the epic Mahabharata, is the song of the Lord Krishna to Arjuna, a mighty warrior, who is about to go into battle against his brothers and is feeling overwhelmed with sorrow at the futility of war.

The first of the three stages of meditation is:

VI. *Dharana* (concentration)

You say, 'White Eagle, you tell us to control our thoughts—but it is not possible!'

I will give you a simple exercise. When you have a piece of work to do, even if it is only hammering a nail into a piece of wood, do it with all your care. Concentrate your whole being on the job in hand. Do not do one thing while thinking about a dozen others. Make yourself interested in the particular piece of work in hand. How often do you listen to a conversation and absorb nothing? The conversation may seem to you to be futile–but perhaps you are the foolish one. Forget everything else but your companion as you are conversing with him.... Take this very seriously, because it offers a practical and simple method of thought control. Centre your whole attention on what you are doing, always.

White Eagle, THE GENTLE BROTHER

How often are we ever totally *with* what we are doing, instead of letting the mind wander on to what comes next, worrying about tomorrow, attached to the past, flitting hither and thither?

Being totally in the Now, in the moment, totally with whatever we are doing, is the first stage of meditation: that is, concentration.

We can do this just in our daily life, in whatever tasks are ours, yet we can see that it does not come that easily. But the concentration required for the *asanas* and *pranayama* helps very much to bring this centredness in whatever we do. So when we start our meditation we can concentrate on one point—whether that be on our breath, the light in our heart, the steady flame of a candle, a beautiful flower, or saying a mantra such as the *Om*. The *Om* is an ancient mantra meaning All, the sound from the beginning of time, the sound that brought the universe into being. It is the omnipotent, the omnipresent, which when chanted takes us to the heart of our being, where all is one.

To be able really to concentrate requires regular practice. As a start, take just ten minutes at the end of a gentle posture and relaxation and breathing session, as the mind and body are then prepared to concentrate. Do not be concerned if you feel unable to get anywhere or see anything, or unable to get away from busy thoughts. It may not seem that you are achieving anything, but the reason we feel this is precisely that we are used to being busy, getting results, 'doing'. Just sitting regularly and being content with this will have an effect on your whole being, your whole life. It will bring peace, centredness, contentment, acceptance, vitality, one-pointedness, compassion, understanding, and freedom from pain, anxiety and stress.

Remember you do not have to see visions, have great illuminations or understanding to benefit from meditation. Just practise being with yourself, give yourself this time each day to watch, and observe without judgment. Watch the mind when it intrudes, as it inevitably will; watch the thoughts, but do not get wrapped up in them, do not follow them, just observe them come and go and then bring your awareness back to the point of your concentration. If you are not sure what to concentrate on just watch your breath come and go; be in your heart. At the end, if you want to, bring in an affirmation given in the *yamas* and *niyamas* or one of your own choosing: the end of a meditation is the most powerful time to use an affirmation.

The second stage is:

VII. *Dhyana* (contemplation)

Endeavour to find yourself, the real 'I' beneath the outer coats of flesh and mind which obscure it. To do this try to think in terms of three; first, think of the ordinary person that you are in daily life; next, think about the soul, known only to yourself (or so you think); and thirdly, try to find the place of stillness and quiet at the centre of your being, the real 'I'.

As you learn to withdraw into your inner self, the outer self will, as it were, dissolve; and the inner self begin to assert itself. This inner self is a personality, a soul—and a something more. If you will train yourself in contemplation, you will find that beneath the soul there is a place of stillness, of blankness, of nothingness if you like. Yet when you are confronted with the seeming nothingness which lies beneath the conscious self, you will gradually become aware of an all-ness, a sense of affinity with universal life and at-one-ment with God. In this condition there can be no separation, no darkness, no fear: nothing exists but love and an exquisite joy which permeates your whole being.

White Eagle, GOLDEN HARVEST

When our flow of concentration is uninterrupted and we can just be with whatever we are concentrating on, then we are in a state of contemplation. This is often likened to water taking the shape of the container it is in. The mind becomes the object on which it is concentrating, there is no separation. This state cannot be forced or brought about by our will, it is given, it just comes naturally, unexpectedly, out of our concentration. There are days, weeks even, when it may seem to us that it does not come at all. This does not mean that we have failed. On another occasion it may come by surprise, at times such as when we feel at one with nature—watching a beautiful sunset, swimming in the sea, sitting in a green meadow—or when we feel at one with another person in a heart-to-heart communication, in making love; or when we are at one with whatever we are doing, reading, writing, being a mother or father, or holding a tiny baby—one with our work or pleasure. In meditation, it can be a moment of timelessness, of total absorption, of total peace and fulfilment of joy.

On other occasions, our meditations can feel rather laborious and unfruitful, but the effect is then felt at other times of the day, so do not be concerned if you do not feel this total absorption: be patient and unattached to the desire for it.

The third stage is:

VIII. *Samadhi* (oneness, bliss)

Meditation helps souls to expand in the consciousness of God. And then again there are souls who have been prepared for aeons past for this conscious union with God. There comes a moment when suddenly all barriers go, and that soul is for a flash (or longer) conscious of itself and God and conscious of the whole universe. It is conscious that it is one with 'THAT'; that it is part of 'THAT'; that there is no separation from 'THAT' and there is no separation from any affinity; it is all in all and complete in 'THAT', the Indivisible.

From a White Eagle teaching

Truly, Brahman is Life itself
shining through all beings.
Knowing It the wise can talk of nothing else.
And he who

swimming in the bliss of the Self,
   delighting in its play,
   still enjoys a life of action,
He is the greatest of those who know Brahman.

When the mind and body have been purified
   through meditation, through Truth,
   through understanding and simplicity,
Then the perfected behold the Self,
   pure and brilliant....

The mind is kept ever active by the senses.
When they have withdrawn
   and the mind become still,
Then the subtle Self shines forth.

When the mind rests steady and pure,
   then whatever you desire
         those desires are fulfilled,
   and whatever you think of
         those thoughts materialise.
So, you who desire good fortune
revere the knower of the Self.

He who knows the Self
   knows the supreme abode of Brahman,
   in which the universe lies resplendent.

MUNDAKA UPANISHAD

Samadhi is the ultimate state in meditation, the experience of complete bliss, rapture, at-one-ment with our Higher Self, with God, with Brahman. It is given by the grace of God, out of our aspirations, out of our yearning to return to the centre from whence we came, out of at-one-ment with our Higher Self.

It comes in a flash of illumination; and once experienced, even just for an instant, there is a yearning to return there. We can if we choose be constantly in that state, even in strife or chaos—we can take ourselves out of separation and know union, oneness with the Divine in ourselves, wherever we are, whatever we are doing.

The word 'THAT' is not an entirely satisfactory translation—

we simply do not have the words in English—but it is used in many yoga texts. We can easily say about *samadhi*, '*Neti, Neti*'—meaning it is not THAT, nor is it *THAT*, and yet it is impossible to put into words what 'THAT' is, it has to be experienced, to be felt, to be lived, yet we are It. As the father explains to his son, Svetaketu, in the Chandogya Upanishad:

When the bees collect the nectar from many different plants, blending them all into one honey, the individual nectars no longer think, 'I come from this plant', 'I come from that plant'. In the same way, my son, all creatures when they contact Being lose all awareness of their individual natures. But when they return from Being they regain their individuality. Whether tiger, or lion, or wolf, or boar, or worm, or fly, or gnat, or even mosquito, they become themselves again.

And that Being which is the subtlest essence of everything, the supreme reality, the Self of all that exists, THAT ART THOU, Svetaketu....

All rivers, whether they flow to the East or to the West, have arisen from the sea and will return to it again. Yet once these rivers have merged with the sea they no longer think, 'I am this river', 'I am that river'. In the same way, my son, all these creatures, when they merge again with Being, do not remember that they originally arose from Being and wound their individual ways through life.

Now that Being which is the subtlest essence of everything, the supreme reality, the Self of all that exists, THAT ART THOU, Svetaketu....

If you were to chop at the root of this great tree, it would bleed but it would not die. If you were to chop at its trunk, it would bleed but it would not die. If you were to chop at its branches, it would bleed but it would not die. Permeated by sap, its life energy, the tree stands firm, drinking and enjoying its nourishment.

But if the sap withdraws from one of the branches then that branch withers. If it withdraws from a second branch then that branch withers. If it withdraws from a third branch then that branch also withers. If the sap withdraws from the whole tree then the whole tree withers and dies. In just the same way, my son, when the Self withdraws from the body the body dies, though the Self lives on.

And that Being which is the subtlest essence of everything, the supreme reality, the Self of all that exists, THAT ART THOU, Svetaketu.

CHANDOGYA UPANISHAD, Chapter VI

Samadhi is the realization that THAT ART THOU: in other words, pure being.

CHAPTER TWO

The Chakras

The central chakra is the heart centre. When this power is released in the individual it should go forth from the heart in love…. It must go through the heart for safe use; it must go forth from the heart, as Jesus the Christ directed, in great compassion, in selfless love. All people who have developed the heart chakra and are in the habit of loving their fellow beings, loving animals, loving nature, loving to give out love, are healers giving the most vital and the greatest healing power that can be given to the world through love.

From a White Eagle teaching

THIS SECTION is not easy to write, although there are a lot of different theories and ideas about the chakras, for unless the chakras mean something subjectively to us, the theories do not amount to very much. It is better, therefore, to think about how we can become aware of the chakras rather than to do a lot of hard thinking about them.

We are all aware of instinctive feelings when we talk about 'gut feelings', or 'gut reactions' to someone or some situation. That awareness comes from the lower energy centres around the navel and solar plexus. A strong emotional feeling or reaction comes from the energy centres around the solar plexus, while a heart-felt feeling of love and compassion can be felt around the heart area.

Greater awareness of this subtle energy system that co-exists with the physical system comes through the practice of yoga and meditation. We become more aware of the reactions in the energies of our own body to situations and people

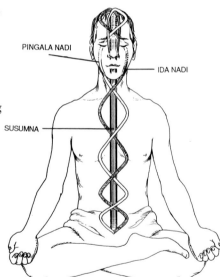

PINGALA NADI

IDA NADI

SUSUMNA

around us. We become aware of where there are blocks in the energy and feel the yoga practice gradually free those blocks. But if there is no awareness of the chakras to start with, do not be concerned; nor (if you can) sceptically dismiss them entirely, for when your body develops this awareness, then that will be the time to consider them in more depth.

The subtle and inner flow of energy in our bodies has been mentioned in the *asana* section, where it is described as being either of the sun or masculine type or of the moon or feminine type, the two being balanced in the perfect body.

As the diagram shows, there are channels for the energy, known as *nadis*. The channel which comes from the lunar, feminine energy is called the *ida*, and it starts in the left nostril, moves to the crown of the head and then descends, moving backwards and forwards across the spine to the base. The channel which carries the solar, masculine energy is called the *pingala*: it starts in the right nostril, moves to the crown of the head, and then backwards and forwards down across the spine to the base. At certain points along the spine (and in the head), the *nadis* connect to *kosas* or sheaths that enclose the soul in the body, the sheaths which White Eagle refers to in his teaching as the etheric body, the causal body, and so on. Here we use the Sanskrit names, but they equate quite easily to the 'bodies' he describes. Where the *nadis* and *kosas* connect are the chakras. They are like vortices or flywheels of rotating energy from which we can give out or take in energy, feelings and intuitions from others and the world around us.

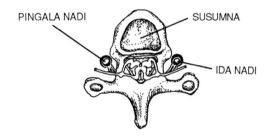

PINGALA NADI   SUSUMNA

IDA NADI

The main chakras, but not the only ones, are:

MULADHARA CHAKRA
(*mula*, root, source; *adhara*, support, vital part)

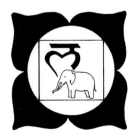

The base or root centre is situated at the base of the spine, the coccyx bone, and is the centre which earths us, grounds us; connects us to Divine Mother and mother earth. It is the seat of the earth element. It has to do with our survival, our will to be, our power, confidence, self-acceptance, vitality and strength. If this centre is blocked, then it is owing to fear of being in the world and difficulties in any of these areas. When it is activated it gives tremendous vitality, and the ability to sublimate sexual desire. The sheath encasing the soul here is the *annamaya kosa* or anatomical sheath of nourishment.

SVADHISTHANA CHAKRA
(*sva*, vital force, soul; *adhisthana*, seat or abode)

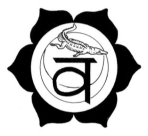

The sacral centre, situated at the level of the sacrum, the 'sacred bone' in the pelvis, connects to the organs of generation, the gonads and the endocrine glands associated with the gonads. It is the centre connected with the water element. This centre is connected to our sexuality or sensitivity, our feelings of attraction to others and to the world around and to our sense of security, self-esteem, personal creativity and social behaviour-patterns. Blocks in the sacral centre are due to a feeling that any of these areas are threatened. When it is activated, we become free from disease, vibrantly healthy, friendly and compassionate.

MANIPURAKA CHAKRA
(*manipura*, navel)

The nervous plexus is situated at the navel and is the seat of the

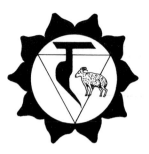

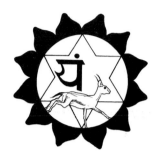

fire element. When it is brought to life we can remain calm in all circumstances. The *svadisthana* and the *manipuraka* chakras are the base of the *pranamaya kosa*, the physiological body, connected to the lower internal organs, the blood and the glands. Both these chakras are involved in *pranayama*.

SURYA CHAKRA
(*surya*, sun)

The solar plexus is situated at the level of the diaphragm and connects to the lungs, the breathing, the kidneys and the adrenal glands (just above the kidneys). This centre relates us to our environment, to people and to things; it draws in energy and lets out stress. It has to do with the expression 'gut feelings' and with possessive love and dependent love. A block in the solar plexus is due to our feeling threatened in the areas mentioned and anything 'out in the world'. When this centre is open we are able to take light and vitality in from the sun, creating a link to the higher worlds giving us a broader, more compassionate vision of our immediate environment.

ANAHATA CHAKRA
(*anahata*, unbeaten)

This is the heart centre, situated at the level of the heart on the spine. It is connected to our heart-felt feelings, our love for others, for God, for the world. It is the balance point in the centres and the focal point for opening and developing—as long as the heart centre remains open, all the others are safe and protected. It has to do with the whole: holistic thinking, unconditional love, healing, humility, responsibility, goodwill, tolerance, empathy, compassion and vulnerability. Blocks in this centre derive from lack of emotional security, from protecting ourselves against the recurrence of past hurts—which will in fact recur all the time we hold onto the fear and continue to block this centre.

The difference between the feeling of the solar plexus and the heart centre is that the solar plexus is selective, and inwardly determines what you are seeing out there; for it is linked to our inbuilt belief system about ourselves and about the world as we see it. The heart, by contrast, picks up the soul quality of a person: it sees what actually 'is' rather than a coloured point of view. So it is all-inclusive and non-judgmental.

Through the constant practice of yoga there develops an awareness of more and more chakras besides these main ones. Mr Iyengar gives an extra chakra, the *manas* ('individual mind') chakra, between the solar plexus and the heart. It links these two chakras and is the seat of the emotions involved in the heart and the solar plexus. The balance between these two is brought about by *pranayama*, where retention of the breath is involved.

The *manas* and the *anahata* chakra form the basis for the *manomaya kosa*—the psychological sheath. When stimulated, it strengthens and stabilizes the heart centre, freeing us from the desire for sensual pleasures, so that we are willingly desirous of the spiritual path, but not inclined to force it.

VISUDDHA CHAKRA
(visuddha, pure)

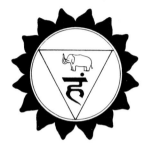

The throat centre is situated in the body at the level of the throat and is connected with the vocal cords, the thyroid gland and the neck. It is related to the ether element. It is known as the trust centre, for it governs our sense of trust in ourselves and in others, in the Universe, in the process of life. It holds our self-expression, our individuality and our desire for peace.

We block this centre if we are not willing to compromise, will not communicate with others and do not trust. The throat centre is the basis for the *vijnanamaya kosa*—the intellectual body. When it is opened, our power of understanding develops.

AJNA CHAKRA
(ajna, command)

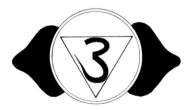

This is the brow centre. Situated in the centre of the forehead and known as the third eye, it is connected to the brain, the vision and the pituitary gland (the pituitary gland is the master gland which controls and compensates for all the other glands in the endocrine system.) It has to do with outward control, self-control, ambition, choices, telepathy, assertiveness, planning. We block this centre if any of these things cause us difficulty. When freed, we gain control over all the other *kosas* or sheaths. As this sheath is the *anandamaya kosa*—the abode of joy—we become truly full of joy for life.

SAHASRARA CHAKRA
(sahasrara, thousand)

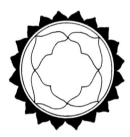

The crown centre—the thousand-petalled lotus—flowers at the crown when the energy rises right up the spine from the base to the crown. It is connected to the pineal gland. This centre is our connection to the universe, and through it we can truly feel children of the universe. It is open and active, according to yoga philosophy, from birth to seven years. When there is trauma, a breaking off of our connection to the universe, this centre is affected. It is especially liable to be affected up to the time we are seven years old. Many of us have seen pictures of Vietnamese and Cambodian refugee children with their hands over their crown, rocking backwards and forwards in an attempt to comfort themselves. It also has to do with transpersonal awareness, inner development and unity in all things. This centre is blocked if we feel cut off or cut ourselves off from the world and feel real aloneness. When freed we feel one with all life, one with the universe, one with the supreme Spirit.

All the centres have their link to the physical body via the endocrine system, the ductless glands. Physically, the centres are situated at a point on the spine at the back of the body. Seen from the front, they appear to have opened out and are to be visualized a little lower down than they are at the back, except for the brow and crown centres. They are like flowers of light that can open and close depending on how we are feeling. It is at these centres that we sense, feel and pick up conditions from our surroundings or from other people.

Healing is given through these centres. Disease is the result of a clogging or blockage of them, and pouring light of different colours in through the centres at the etheric level clears them. This works through to the outer physical or emotional disturbance, restoring health.

The more we practise yoga the more aware of the centres and the energy flow we become, and the more we tend to unblock and clear them. As long as we have a balance between strength and suppleness, the body will have the strength to take this awareness and sensitivity and yet still be 'in the world'.

In yoga philosophy the back of the body is known as the West of the body: it is strong and bony, more entrenched in matter, more connected to the nurturing mother principle of the earth. The front of the body is the East: it is softer, more yielding and able to open to the light, to the sun, connected to the masculine principle, that of going forward to meet life. If we keep the back of the body strong, particularly through the standing postures and the inverted postures, then the front of the body will be able to open to the light, which is the effect of meditation and of the back-bending and hip-opening postures. When there is imbalance between the two we can feel over-sensitive to the world around us, particularly to noise and crowds, or feel as though we are picking up negative influences. Yet it is not helpful to blame the world

outside. If we look inside and stand strong and firm in our physical bodies, centred in the light, we can take any battering that the world seems to give us. What is without us is a reflection of what is within us and we cannot hide away from it.

As well as the *ida* and the *pingala*, there is a central main channel that carries energy, called the *susumna*. It runs from the base of the spine through the spinal column, meeting the centres as it goes. At the base of the spine there is the feminine energy coiled up and likened to a serpent asleep, the *kundalini*. *Kundalini* means coiled female serpent: it is the divine cosmic energy also known as the *shakti* energy. In Indian legend Shakti is the consort of the Lord Shiva. Shiva unintentionally pierces her with his third eye when he is in deep meditation, whereupon she dies as Shakti and reincarnates as Parvati and reunites with Shiva. Shiva resides in the brow centre, the third eye, and he represents the masculine energy and the Higher Self, the God Self. Shakti being pierced by Shiva and dying is symbolic of the outer self or the ego falling away to be reborn, so that reunion with Shiva is the union of the outer earthly self with the inner, Higher Self.

So while there is this interchange of masculine and feminine energies from the right to the left side of the body through the centres, there is a polarization through the centre with the base and the crown. Through yoga, meditation, both of them ways of developing spiritual awareness and thus creating a balance in the right side of the brain and the body, the feminine energy in the base awakens and rises up the *susumna*, the central column, towards the crown, to meet the masculine energy, residing in the brow. Yoga is said to balance the subconscious mind in the base centres with the conscious mind in the head and the meeting place is in the heart. So if we can centre ourselves in the heart chakra, operating, working, living, and thinking with 'the mind in the heart', we can draw Shiva down from the head to meet Shakti in the heart in the divine cosmic marriage, the 'mystical marriage'.

There is a great deal said about the dangers of drawing the *kundalini* energy up. In the various practices that do this before the body is ready for it, what actually happens is that *kundalini* is irritated, awoken too soon, and she lashes out uncontrollably. Many things can have this effect—hard drugs, heavy rock music, forcing the body too soon into the Lotus pose, rocking around on the base of the spine. They create a terrific disturbance in the base and this is sometimes manifested as strong sexual energy. Similarly, through certain brow-centre meditations the *kundalini* can actually be drawn up to the brow to create a strong sense of one's own power. The person then wants to take over the world, to dominate and control; thinks himself or herself all-powerful.

However, if we are always centred in the heart, consciously withdrawing from the head mind, and at the same time maintaining the stability and strength to stand firm on the earth, there is no danger in spiritual unfoldment; and the practice of the *asanas* gives us this stability. The energy and energy centres can gradually, gently become awakened, bringing about an opening of the heart—the balance point—particularly. The energy can then safely be drawn up, illuminating and energizing us, freeing us from heaviness.

As we become aware of these subtle internal energies we can gradually bring them under our control. If we feel very vulnerable or that our energy is draining out of us, the feeling often comes from the solar plexus and the base centre, and we can consciously contain and direct the energy. If the solar plexus feels vulnerable, consciously draw your energy in and see it circulating around the whole trunk area: see the solar plexus just closing, a little like a flower at night. Seal the solar plexus with an equal-sided cross of light upon it and circle it in light. If your energy feels to be draining out of the base, take your awareness there and see the energy circulating around inside the pelvis and then coming back up again. You can seal this centre too. We can also direct the energy ourselves to any organ or part of the body that needs help, although it is often more effective for someone else to put their hands on the place, as the energy can then flow from one to the other, helping both participants. During healing, however, the consciousness always remains in the heart centre. So in yoga practice, and in meditation and daily life, one can be conscious of this movement of energy, and of coming down to the heart, out of the head mind; centred in the love of the heart, able to give and receive love whatever the circumstances.

There is a beautiful saying in the Rig Veda, one of the most ancient Hindu writings:

> If you get close to the fire of Parvati, that burns away the chaff and leaves the pure essence of being … do not go up to the mountain! Go to the market place and trade … and … fall in love!

This balance and interchange of masculine and feminine energies within ourselves also reflects and relates to those with whom we come closely into contact in the world. This is most important, as it is no help to humanity if we are all so 'spiritual' and 'up in the clouds' that we cannot relate to our brothers and sisters on the earth. So balancing and harmonizing the energies within ourselves through the practice of yoga will help us to improve our relationships with other people.

This is the most important thing on earth. Our reason for being here is to enable us to open our hearts in love to all around us and all on the planet—whether male, female, black, white, animal or plant—and to the earth itself.

CHAPTER THREE

Notes on the Practice of Yoga

You must have courage for your work; courage to heal, to comfort; courage to give service, and courage never to doubt God's power, or the power of God to work through you. To think you are no good is to doubt God's power. Of yourself you are merely a channel, but that which dwells in you, the power of God, is the directing, controlling, creative principle in life.

White Eagle, THE GENTLE BROTHER

IT IS SAID that we are beginners in yoga for the first twenty years of practice! Therefore a great deal of perseverance is required, and we may not become aware of the effects for some considerable time, particularly the inner effects talked about in the *yamas* and the *niyamas* and the opening of the centres. The crucial time for many people seems to be after two or three years. Often after this we either go into yoga for life or stop completely. Once we are on this path for life we are totally committed to working, developing and evolving ourselves; yet not for ourselves, but for the upliftment of humanity.

When you start on the postures, it may be difficult to see that what appears to be a series of physical exercises can have such a far-reaching effect. To me they are not exercises at all but sacred, spiritual movements of the inner and outer body that attune us to our source. Do not worry if you do not feel this for the first few years of practice, for this awareness gradually develops as we centre ourselves in our hearts and let go the busy head mind.

In the descriptions of the postures, I have often used words like 'lift', 'spread', 'open'. When this instruction is given, take your awareness inwards and see the lifting, spreading, opening coming with the breath. These are internal feelings that come with practice rather than outer movements that are precisely describable. So, for example, in lifting the chest do not be tempted to lift yourself by your shoulders and the outer body but feel an internal lift through the centre under the breast-bone. If you do not feel that inner lift at first, imagine it and then it will in time come naturally. If you are in the habit, as many of us are, of hunching your shoulders and caving your chest in, then it is going to take some while of continued practice to lift and open it out.

More specific outer movements such as taking the top rim of the pelvis (iliac crest) back do come from the internal movement of spreading the belly back into the pelvis and stretching the base of the spine down towards the ground. But again it is the internal awareness and concentration that brings these movements and the connection of the mind to that part of the body.

The Inner and Outer Bodies

You will see that there are many references in this book to the inner and outer bodies. This is a concept I learned to work with from my two inspiring teachers Angela Farmer and Victor Van Kooten. Anyone who has attended their courses will have gained a deep feeling for the inner and outer bodies; and learnt how they move with one another and how the inner body can lift out of the outer body, how the outer body can let go of its hold upon the inner. My personal understanding is as follows:

The outer body relates to the outer self and to the 'mind in the head' (as opposed to the 'mind in the heart'). It is the physical part that is entrenched in matter and holds all our fears, our worries, our tension, our responsibility and our strain. For example, tightness and tension in the shoulders is created by a feeling of the burdens of life. We carry all our worries and responsibility—the weight of the world—on our shoulders, hence the tension. If we lift ourselves up with the inner body, by the trust in God which the heart centre naturally holds, we can see what a waste of energy worry is and literally drop the burden off our shoulders; telling the outer body, the outer self, to relax its hold on us.

Ask your higher wisdom
if it is not true that without worry,
you would have arrived exactly where you are now,
and more pleasantly.

Doubt is the rabbit's foot of fear.

Worry and fear are not tickets on the express train.
They are extra baggage.
You were going that way anyway.

EMMANUEL'S BOOK II: THE CHOICE FOR LOVE

The inner body relates to the inner self: the subconscious, situated in the base centres; the flow of subtle energy, through the spine and round the organs. It also relates to the 'mind in the heart'. White Eagle talks about the 'eternal body'; this seems to me to be close to the yogic concept of the inner body. It is the inner body also that is sensitive to internal movements of energy as well as to the external energy interchange in the atmosphere, in other people, and in groups and societies.

For example, you will notice that there are references in the postures to the movement of the belly. This is different from the abdomen and refers to the whole cavity of the pelvis, and most importantly the energy-flow in that area. In order to move the belly, we need to move our consciousness out of our heads and be centred down in the body. At the beginning of our practice we tend to lead with the head, just as we tend in daily life to operate from our heads, and so the postures become forced and strained—the ego will be uppermost, pushing us as far as we can into the posture. It is not the final achievement of the posture that matters but the journey to get there and the awareness developed on the way; so there is no need to perform fancy poses or hurry into difficult ones. It is not a performance—a performance is ego-based—nor is it necessary to force the body: say, to take the head down in forward bends, losing all awareness. A straight, stretched spine has far more awareness in it than a spine that is curved by dropping the head, which would be to allow the head to lead.

Suppose we do nothing but the Mountain pose. If this is done with perfect awareness in every part of the body, then the others are not needed; although conversely the other postures do help to bring perfect poise to the Mountain pose.

To develop perfect awareness we need to be centred in the heart and in the body. If we bring our awareness down into the base and into the belly the initial impetus to move into the posture comes from there, and there will then be far more internal movement and life in the posture. We can, if we choose, force the outer body into the postures. For example, in the hip movements such as the Cobbler, we can push on the knees; but they immediately spring back and actually tighten even more in reaction to being forced, whereas if we let go and spread in the belly, this releases the tightly-held sacrum bone so that the thigh-bones can release their hold into the hips. The inner body can then lift up out of the hips into the heart area, giving us that light-hearted feeling that comes from extending fully into the postures without straining.

So awareness of the inner body and the belly are important in the postures. Yet do not always expect to feel this at first, for there needs to be an initial breaking-down of the armour of the outer body: an armour we have built up around us from child-hood to protect ourselves from hurt. When we strengthen the inner body and lift ourselves up from our centre to connect to our source of light; when we trust in the process of life, then we no longer need this protective armour, and it can fall away, leaving the light, open, inner body full of love and trust.

Good and Bad Pain

The course of human life is like that of a great river which, by the force of its own swiftness, takes quite new and unforeseen channels where before there was no current—such varied currents and unpremeditated changes are part of God's purpose for our lives.

Life is not an artificial canal to be confined within prescribed channels.

When once this is clearly seen in our lives, then we shall not be able to be misled by any mere fabrications.

Rabindranath Tagore

Yoga teachers are often asked if we need to feel pain in the postures to produce any results. The answer to this is that there are two types of pain. When we begin to change and develop ourselves, to move on in our lives from where we have been up to this point, there is resistance from the ego, for it does not want to let go of its strong hold. This manifests in the outer body as tightly held muscles and ligaments. So when we move a muscle that has not been used for a very long time, it feels as if there is quite a resistance to the movement. The stretch, however, actu-ally feels very releasing and relaxing, and it is known as good pain. It stops when you stop doing the posture.

If in any posture a sharp, stabbing pain arises, or there is a sharp reaction in the muscles or bones to moving into a posture or a pain that does not go away once you have stopped doing the posture, then this is bad pain. It is caused by a local weakness and by over-extension. It indicates that you are doing the posture in an unhealthy and therefore harmful way for you. If there is a weakness in one spot, there is a counterbalancing tightness and tension in another part of the body. For example, sciatica in one side of the sacrum is generally actually caused by the other side of the sacrum and the whole hip joint being comparatively tighter and tenser there than the painful side. So work more on the opposite side, particularly in standing postures and forward bends, and this will actually relieve the painful side. The painful side needs to be relaxed and rested, and the tight side needs to be worked and released.

Similarly, if there is over-extension in one part, there is counterbalancing or tightness in the opposite part. For example, the hamstring muscles that insert into the buttock-bone run right down the backs of the legs and insert into the calf-bone, and often become over-extended. This can be seen in those who lock the knees back, which in turn creates too much curvature in the back: an inward curve in the lumbar spine and an outward one in the neck. The corresponding complex set of muscles on the front of the thigh bone, inserting into the hip and knee joint, where we hold a lot of emotion, will be tightly-held, hard and tense. So we work on these front thigh muscles, by allowing the knees to feel a little bent in such postures as *uttanasana* or *trikonasana*. The legs do eventually need to be straight but if we have been over-bending them backwards, the only way to get them straight is to bend them a corresponding amount forwards, then lift from the buttock-bones to straighten the leg. The knee will feel bent for some time before we learn to connect to the muscle that will straighten it without locking it. Eventually this will bring the front thigh-muscles to life—*supta virasana* and back bends will also bring a great deal of awareness to these muscles and release much tension held there. This takes quite a bit of practice, so do persevere!

Awareness of good pain and bad pain gradually helps you to bring life to all parts of the body, by your becoming conscious of which parts 'give' too much, are lazy, or where there is no 'give' at all: these are tense. By taking your awareness down into your body, you learn how to balance them out.

Pain and tension felt in the body is actually a message to the mind that something needs doing, something needs changing. The body has had enough abuse and is rebelling—so pain is actually your teacher, your saviour.

Where there is pain, there is resistance to change, to surrender of the ego, to trust in the universe, in God.

Often the posture which seems to create pain and discomfort is actually the posture which will alleviate and eventually cure the problem. For example, *supta virasana* and *baddha konasana* (in the seated posture section, chapter 9) are given as a cure for varicose veins. It seems as though bending the knees is the last thing that would help if veins are swollen. However, if we did these postures as part of a proper programme, first inverting the legs up the wall or in Shoulder-stand for five to ten minutes, and then stretching the legs well, by the time we then did *supta virasana* and *baddha konasana* on a lift of blocks or cushions, they would feel very beneficial.

In any neck problem or problem of high or low blood pressure, the best advice is not to do inverted postures. Done in the normal way these would aggravate the problem, although a skilled teacher could teach them in such a way that they would cure the problem over a period of time.*

If a posture does create pain or does not feel beneficial you need to find an alternative way of doing it. Do study the points to watch that are given with each posture in this book. Also use your own awareness, for if we work from the ego, the outer self, without awareness, we tend to block subtle releases and reinforce inheld tension, and that creates pain.

It is often helpful to ask the body what is required or ask the Higher Self. There is a technique that could be useful here called focusing (from a book called FOCUSSING by Gene Gendlin). If ever I do not know what to do for a pupil or what would help them best then I ask God, or my Higher Self. It does not matter who you think you are asking, just ask and wait. This has never failed me. Often I immediately get a picture of a posture, or an alternative way of doing a posture which they could use to help themselves; sometimes it comes afterwards, when I or the person concerned are ready to hear it.

* This would need a good teacher and is not advisable on your own. However, anyone is welcome to write to the publishers of this book or to come for a day or two to classes (see 'Useful Addresses' at the back), or have a private lesson if they do not have a teacher and would like some personal help.

Unevenness in the Postures

The problem of unevenness has already been mentioned in the section in 'The eight limbs of yoga' on *asanas*, in connection with the right and left side of the body. At different stages in our practice of yoga, there often comes tremendous awareness of unevenness and difference between the two sides of the body. This can feel very awkward and uncomfortable for a time, especially in *tadasana*, the Mountain pose.

This is in fact a very good stage, for in it we are actually just becoming aware of a difference or imbalance that has existed since early childhood, when we were taught, or learnt by copying, to use one side more than or differently from the other. Stay with the awareness of unevenness and awkwardness because even the awareness will go a long way towards balancing them out. It is also helpful to use a full-length mirror or to have your back against the wall or bannisters. This helps you to work more evenly on each side by seeing or feeling where the tightness is.

As I have shown, it can be very helpful to go to the stiffer, tighter side an extra time or to stay there a little longer to bring a greater awareness to it. It is said that yoga would eventually make us ambidextrous! I have personally noticed this in myself and others. So be aware in your daily life how much more reliant you are on one side than the other; and in little tasks, such as picking things up and cleaning the teeth, just try bringing the other side in more. In this way you will greatly increase the sense of balance between the two sides of the body, and between the head mind, the heart mind and the body mind and in life generally so as to bring greater integration of the whole self on all levels.

Using the Sanskrit Names

Sanskrit is the root and oldest member of all Indo-European languages. Latin itself derives from Sanskrit. The word 'sanskrit' literally means 'that which has been adorned, decorated or transformed' and is usually translated as 'the perfected'.

The Sanskrit words for the terms in the postures and the philosophy have been used, and a translation given, because just the feeling of the word conveys a great deal of the meaning of the term or posture at a deep inner level, even if the outer self finds them difficult or impossible to remember. So try saying the Sanskrit to yourself and out loud. This will obviously be much easier if you have actually heard it spoken in a class or on tape but if not do still study the words.

The Sanskrit names of the postures are given in transliteration here, with accentual marks omitted. Because they are western transliterations, they are in most cases pronounced roughly as they would sound in English, but the following notes may be helpful:

• The first 'a' in *asana* is long as in 'path' and the stress falls on this syllable. Otherwise, 'a' is usually short, as in 'mat'; 'ar' is

long, as in 'part'. The final 'a' in *asana* is usually not pronounced, although practice does vary in different parts of India. Thus *tadasana* will generally be pronounced 'tad-arsan'.

• An 'h' after a double 'tt', as in *utthita*, after a 'b', as in *virabhadrasana*, after a 'd', as in *baddha*, is lightly aspirated, but does not affect the preceding consonant: e.g., 'utt-hita', 'virab-hadrasana'.

• In *parivrtta* and *vrksasana* a short 'i' is sounded after the 'r' where there is no vowel in the transliteration, so that the words sound roughly 'parivritta', 'vriksasana'.

The Sanskrit words all have an inner meaning and an outer meaning, as has been explained in various places. For example, *danda* means staff or stick at the outer level, and at the inner level it means authority—to authorize, to bring into being, to originate. The postures can work at both levels if we allow them to do so, if we let go of the idea that they are merely physical exercises and tune into the beautiful movement and awareness that they bring.

Sanskrit words are also interesting when they are split up, as we saw with the word *hatha*, in the *asana* section. Another example of this is the word *guru*: as one word, it means spiritual teacher, spiritual preceptor, one to devote oneself and one's life to, mentor. Splitting the word up, *gu* means darkness and *ru* means light. This gives a further depth to the word *guru*, in its contradictory meaning: the paradox shows how we need a balance of light and darkness for how could we see where we are if it were not for shadows? A *guru* is one who illumines the darkness.

Breathing in the Postures

All that yoga breathing involves is simply to breathe! Watch that you are not holding your breath, straining to force the air in or pushing it out. Relax, let go, lift up on the inhalation, and move into the posture on an exhalation. Do not hold your breath (and many people do, so constantly be aware) whilst holding the posture. If the breathing is laboured, come up, again exhaling as you move. Inhaling when moving into the posture makes it far more strained. If you exhale as you move, you relax into it much more.

Whilst you are in the posture, spread open on the inhalation, taking the breath into any tightly-held area, and move out of that tightness, extending upwards and outwards with the exhalation.

Inhale when you are ready to come out of the posture; exhale as you move out of it. There is much talk about the necessity for an aerobic effect on the heart and lungs. A criticism of yoga is that it does not give this effect, that the heart rate is not increased, and neither is the breathing rate. This certainly is so in the first stages of practice because the heart, lungs and whole body are gradually being opened out to be able to take a general, moment-by-moment increase of oxygen and life energy to the whole system; whereas many people who go in for aerobics and forceful forms of physical exercise such as jogging to maintain physical fitness start from a point of being very unfit and then suddenly stretch their bodies violently for short lengths of time.

This is a matter of choice, but the violent stretch can be very damaging to the overall balance of the system, especially to the heart, if there is not a high level of fitness, and a general lack of tension in the first place.

If, however, we want to give the system this aerobic effect through yoga, then once we have spent some time on the practice of the standing postures, which are strengthening and make us open, we can go on to practising the *surya namaskar* at a fast pace, jumping from the Dog pose into the standing postures, going up and down in Full arm-balance and back bends at a fast rate. Anybody who has done this in one of Mr Iyengar's classes will certainly know the meaning of an aerobic workout!

Again, personal choice is involved, and do the energetic routine if it feels to be of benefit to you. I occasionally want to do my *asanas* in this way but generally prefer a brisk, long walk for this kind of toning up; it is very complementary to the practice of yoga and is yoga itself when it is performed with awareness.

CHAPTER FOUR

A General Outline of a Programme for the Postures

USUALLY WHEN drawing up your own yoga practice programme, it is better to tune in to your body's needs and feel what it is asking you to do. Simply watch for any tendency always to do the postures that you feel are of no difficulty to you. Have a little go at the ones you do not like so much and you will gradually find that their appeal grows. If you have a day when you need to be told what to do, use one of the three practice tapes I have prepared (see bibliography). Start with the first one if you are new to yoga.

Otherwise, here are some notes to help you devise your own programme.

If you are just starting out on the practice of yoga, start with the first four poses of the standing posture section, chapter 5. Then sit in *virasana*, followed by *baddha konasana*, in the seated postures, chapter 9; then relaxation. After the first two or three weeks, add one standing posture each week; and when you feel ready, start on the forward bend section, chapter 6, working through in the sequence given.

After two or three months of practice, go on to *salamba sarvangasana*, the Shoulder-stand (in the inverted pose section, chapter 8); after one year's practice of Shoulder-stand, go on to the other inverted poses.

After three to six months of practice of the standing postures and the forward-bending postures, go on to the backward-bending and twisting sections (chapters 7 and 11).

After six months of practice go on to the first section of *surya namaskar—svanasana* (the Dog poses, chapter 10). After one year of practice go through the whole of the *surya namaskar*.

For the first five years of practice always go through a section of the standing postures in every practice session to maintain the strength, stability and groundedness. Then vary the others according to your needs. The Dog poses are very beneficial to do every day as they give an overall extension and bring life everywhere. Head- and Shoulder-stands are good to do every day, for the awakening and balance that they bring.

If you need to be woken up, if the body needs to be alert and alive, go through the backward-bending section. If your mind needs to be finely attuned, go through the twisting postures. If you need to be quietened, calmed, and the mind needs some peace, go through the forward-bending section. If you are preparing to meditate or want to relieve tension, go through the seated posture section. If you feel ill, if it's the first day of a period, or if you feel generally run down, practise relaxation and breathing. If you want an overall extension and upliftment, an attunement to the sun, practise the *surya namaskar*.

Generally, take a few postures from each section and vary them day by day. The sequence in which the sections are arranged in this book is chosen to give a balanced, harmonizing order to your practice. So if you are picking one or two from each section, start with the standing postures and work through sequentially. Similarly, if you are wanting to work through one section for the internal effect that type of posture brings, keep to the order given, as they follow on from one another. To me, it feels helpful to do the more dynamic postures in the morning, and the quieter, calmer, forward bends and seated postures in the evening. All the postures given are only a beginning, relatively speaking, yet they do produce overall a balanced effect and are all that you need.

If you feel the need to go further and practise more advanced postures, however, refer to Mr Iyengar's book, LIGHT ON YOGA.

Remember that there is no 'should', 'ought to' or 'cannot' in the practice of yoga, a principle which can be carried over into life. Yoga is more to do with tuning in to what your body, your mind, and indirectly your spirit, wants and needs at a particular time, for this overcomes any inherent laziness and allows us gradually to become aware of the finer, inner tuning and connection between mind, body and spirit. You will gradually find that those things that you feel you cannot do will become possible: you will gain more confidence and movement as you persevere.

One or Two Props which may be Useful

One or two properties are mentioned in the text to help you with the postures.

The best form of chair to use is one with parallel sides, a flat seat and an upright back. Check that the height is just right for you.

A pleated blanket is described for *pranayama* and illustrated below. It is important that it is pleated rather than folded, as this ensures even support either side of the spine. The blocks (right) suggested for support in some of the postures are made of firm plastic foam, which is quite widely available.

Non-slip mats for standing postures, Dog poses, back bends, may be had from many suppliers. In cases of difficulty, they are available from Myron Hobbelen and Glyn Ivens, 4 Felindre Maisonettes, Lon Hendre, Waun Jawr, Aberystwyth, Dyfed SY23 3PY (tel: 0970 611112)

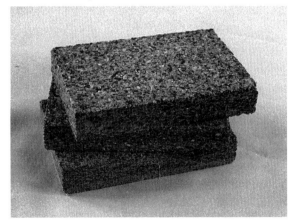

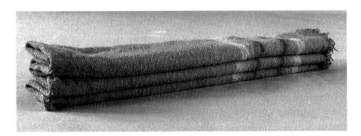

CHAPTER FIVE

Standing Postures

Think for a moment of the difference in your attitude of mind immediately you pull yourself erect and aspire. You seem to be filled with light, and this is exactly what happens when you stand erect, perfectly poised. The spiritual light is able to enter and pass through you without hindrance, to your finger-tips and down your spine to its base; and your feet (free and supple, as they should be) are able to feel and draw magnetism from the earth, and this magnetism circulates through your aura, giving you that vitality and energy for which you long.

It is most important to keep the spine straight, my children, so that the energy of the Sun spirit can pour through the head and descend down the spine.... An erect spine helps to keep the soul in touch with the higher self.

White Eagle, in SUN-MEN OF THE AMERICAS by Grace Cooke

THE STANDING postures are the starting point in the practice of the yoga postures because they bring the firmness and the stability needed to live on the earth—they literally help one to stand easily and strongly. They help one to be more relaxed, steadier and less liable to tiredness. By developing more mobility in the hips, they enable the spine to extend up and out of the hip-joint and sacrum, thereby becoming freer. By bringing life to the feet, the toes, the ball of the foot, the arches, the heels and the ankles, greater independence and efficiency is gained by these units of the body; and together they work to bring increased life-force to the rest of the body by mobilizing the knees and hips, and then in turn helping to open and free the chest. This brings all the subtle energies of the body into a beautiful alignment, enabling the breath to come and go naturally. The feet are said to represent the 'understanding', being under-the-standing; this is the deep, inner understanding and knowing that is at a soul level, rather than at a head level.

The sequence of these standing postures (as with the sequences given in all the chapters) is very important. You do not need to practise them all together, although it is good to do so sometimes as at an inner level they stimulate the chakras or centres (see chapter 2) one by one from the base of the spine to the crown of the head. However, we need always to start with the Mountain to centre us, followed by the Triangle and then the Stretched flank, which will work on the base of the spine and the sacrum: we all tend to be very blocked and tight in these areas, so we need to free and lift the energy from the base upwards. Then some of the others can be left out as long as you keep the overall sequence so that the energy is gradually moving upwards throughout, finishing with either *uttanasana* or *prasarita padottanasana* to bring the balance of the energies from the base to the head and the heart.

You will notice that in the instructions the postures are always given going to the right first, then to the left. This is important to observe in the twists (chapter 11) as the movement then goes with the internal flow of energy from the liver (on the right) clockwise around the body to the spleen (on the left). However, in the postures which stretch the spine straight out to the sides, e.g., *trikonasana* or *parsvakonasana*, it is a good idea to try going to the left first sometimes, as it can bring a deeper awareness of the difference in the two sides and thereby help us to create more balance gradually, through our practice. Also, as explained in Part One, we usually tend to lead with the right side in everyday life, so going to the left first can balance this out.

If you begin to find the postures tiring, relax down into *uttanasana* in between each one, which will refresh and restore you.

AWARENESS AND ATTENTION

Under this heading, which occurs in each of the chapters on the postures, I have wanted to give some feeling of the energy that comes through this group of *asanas*. It is helpful while practising to let your awareness of what your body is doing include this wider dimension as this will help the energy flow through the body, from mind to body and body to spirit.

In each of the standing postures be aware of the firmness of the earth that you are standing on; remember that the energy can come up through the earth through your feet and flow through your body. Feel the crown of the head aspiring to the heavens so that energy can come down from above, from the sun, from pure clear space, joining with the energy of the earth to flow through your body.

Feel the opening, freeing and strengthening of the back, the bony structure of the body on the earth; and the softening and opening of the front of the body, especially the heart centre and the solar plexus, to the incoming energy from the sun.

Tadasana (Mountain Pose)

This posture is so much more than standing straight. It is a conscious awareness, a bringing-to-life of each part of the body, from the firmness of the feet on the ground to the stretching up of the crown of the head to the heavens. The inner body, the spirit, lifts you up through the centre so that the heart can open and free itself from the heaviness of the body, while the rest of the body gradually lets go its hold, its tension.

The feet, stretching down into the ground, are the base of the mountain: firmly planted in matter in order for the spine, and the crown of the head, to extend upward through the clouds heavenwards like the mountain peak. Symbolically the Mountain pose creates a bridge between heaven and earth.

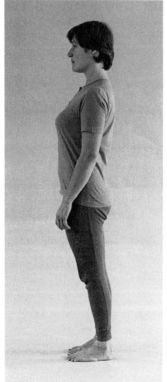 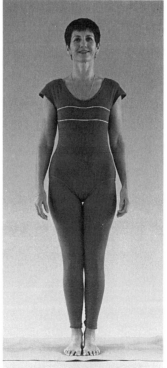

Stand straight with the feet together and in line. If it feels comfortable, have the joints of the big toes and inner ankles just touching; but if you feel unsteady, have the feet a little apart but parallel to each other.

Stretch the big toes forward and towards one another, separating all the toes out, and extend them down into the ground. Feel you can extend up from the outer ankles to the outer hips and from the inner ankles and insteps all the way up the inner legs, keeping the inner heels and joints of the big toes stretching down into the ground.*

Take the backs of the heels firmly down to stretch the backs of the legs. Let the very base of the spine (the coccyx) extend down so that the lumbar spine (the small of the back) can stretch out lengthways and relax back if it tends to push forwards. This will bring the top rim of the pelvis back so that the front of the body lifts up away from the front thighs. Feel the spine lengthen and straighten out as though you are being lifted up from the insteps through to the crown of the head. Then the shoulders can relax down and the chest and heart feel free to lift up. Look straight ahead but without staring. The eyes, face and brain are soft and relaxed.

POINTS TO WATCH AND WORK ON

1. If your hips are uneven or feel uneven, as is the case with a great many people (see chapter 3, pp. 57-58), it will be uncomfortable to have the feet together, so take them far enough apart to be comfortable, but always keep them parallel to one another.

2. When first practising this posture it can be very helpful to stand with the back against a wall or door as a guideline. This also helps you to tuck the base of the spine down and to be aware of where the head and shoulders need to be. Or you can stand in front of a mirror to see if you are straight and even on the right and left sides.

3. Do not push the chest out military-style, but feel that the back and front of the chest can spread evenly, the whole rib-cage spreading to the sides so that the heart and chest can lift without closing in the shoulder blades.

EFFECTS

This posture gradually brings life, awareness and lightness to each part of the body, overcoming the heaviness of gravity, so clearing the mind, making you alert and alive and sensitive to surroundings. It creates an inner balance which brings peace. It relieves backache, neckache and tensions in the shoulders, depression and dullness.

* For an explanation of terms such as 'spread', 'extend', 'open', see chapter 3 (page 54).

Utthita Trikonasana (Triangle Pose)

The triangle is symbolic of the three sides of creation, the triad of Divinity, represented by Brahma, the creator of life, Vishnu, the maintainer, and Shiva, the destroyer of life. The firmness and perfect balance of an equal-sided triangle are reflected in this posture. The feet are firmly grounded in matter, and the rest of the body stretches up and out, the head looking upwards.

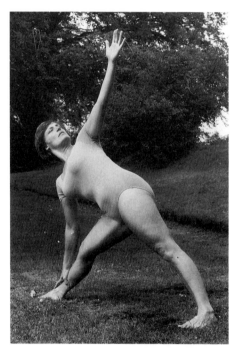

Jump or take the feet three to three-and-a-half feet apart, keeping them in line, and take the arms to the sides at shoulder level. Jumping into the standing postures does bring more 'aliveness' and dynamism, but if this feels at all jarring on the spine or knees, or you prefer to step the feet apart, do so. Stretch down firmly to the outside of the feet, lift the insteps and inner ankles so that you stretch up the inside of the legs. Extend the arms away to the finger-tips and spread the ribs to the side. Then turn the right foot, hip and knee out to the right and the left foot slightly in to the right (illustrated opposite). Inhale, stretch up, lifting the chest a little more; exhale, stretch out and down to the right, from deep in the right hip.

Take the right hand to the right leg or foot, stretching the left hand up. Then try to turn from deep in the right hip up to the left, following that turn all the way along the length of the body so that the ribs and shoulder turn to the ceiling. Finally let the head turn to look up at the left finger-tips, palms forward (main photo, left). While in the pose, stretch the legs and feet firmly down into the ground, rotate the thighs away from one another so that the left hip lifts a little more up and away from the right hip, towards the ceiling. Stay only as long as you feel that you can work and extend into the posture, then inhale and exhale to come up. Inhale, and come back to the centre. Exhaling, turn to the left and repeat on that side. Bring the feet back together on an exhalation.

POINTS TO WATCH AND WORK ON

1. Again it is helpful to use a wall as a guideline, as you are working towards bringing the whole body into a straight line and in one plane, and it can be very difficult to tell if this is so. Being against a wall also helps you to work the hips more.

2. Make sure that you turn not only the foot but the knee and thigh of the front leg. Just to turn the foot puts a strain on the knee, while the hips remain unmoved and tight, making the bend come more from the waist and thus straining the back. The bend should be from the base of the spine so that the whole spine moves to the side to come parallel to the ground.

3. Do not worry to begin with to keep the left hip turned forcefully to the left when moving to the right, as this may just prevent the right hip turning to the right. The left hip can be lifted up and back once you are down in the posture.

4. If the neck feels strained when you turn to look up, it shows you are leading with the head, forcing your body into the posture rather than letting the turn extend gradually out of the base of spine and hips. If so, keep looking forward, the head in line with the chest to begin with; then bring your awareness down to the belly and hips and let the turn come from deep in the right hip. Feel you are turning the right side of the belly up into the left.

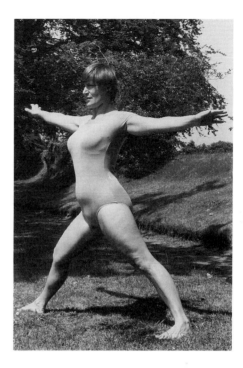

EFFECTS

This posture brings stability and firmness to both body and mind. It strengthens and stretches the limbs and the spine, preventing and relieving arthritis and back problems and toning up the liver and kidneys. Inwardly, it stimulates the centre at the base of the spine, the *muladhara* chakra, the seat of *kundalini* (see chapter 2). Freeing the energy in this very safe, steady way allows us to integrate the energy in the subconscious mind with that in the conscious, head-mind, allowing those energies to meet in the heart. The base centre also has to do with our stability on the earth and with how grounded and comfortable we are in our bodies and on earth. Working in this pose helps us to be grounded, stable and firm on the earth.

Utthita Parsvakonasana (Stretched-flank Pose)

Sanskrit always contains an inner and outer interpretation and meaning. *Parsva* means 'side', but also 'horizon', so by the intense stretch of the side we are extending the fingertips and inwardly our consciousness to the horizon—as far as we can, and then beyond that, continually extending our consciousness to God-consciousness.

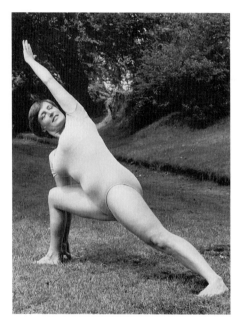

Take the feet four to five feet apart, keeping them in line, and stretching the arms to the side; exhale, extend the arms away out of the shoulders, the legs away out of the hips and down to the feet, firmly spreading the feet out and down into the ground. Turn the right thigh, knee and foot out to the right, the left foot slightly in. Inhale, stretch the spine up out of the hips and lengthen the left thigh out of the hip and stretch down firmly to the outside of the left foot. Exhaling, bend the right knee so that it comes directly above the ankle, with the thigh and shin making a right angle, stretching the right side out to the right. (If the feet are not far enough apart the knee will go right over the foot, creating strain there and in the thigh; or else the thigh will be at an angle to the ground, rather than parallel, creating strain in the hip. Adjust the feet until you can drop right down to bring the

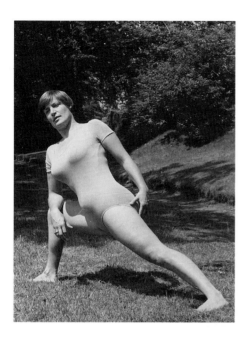

you can extend into it, coming up before the body feels heavy or strained. Inhale as you lift the trunk, and exhaling bring the left foot forward. Repeat the pose to the left. Come back to *tadasana*.

POINTS TO WATCH AND WORK ON

1. With all postures, but particularly these that very much extend the body, only hold the position as long as you can work and extend into it. Come up before you feel heavy or unsteady.

2. Do not let the right knee (when going to the right) roll forward, as this causes the hip to roll outwards and stops the movement coming from the hip-joint.

3. If you have any back problem, or feel dizziness or discomfort, keep the top arm down by the side until this has been corrected, which will happen with continued practice of this and other postures.

EFFECTS

As well as the inner effect of extending the consciousness, this posture strengthens and stabilizes the physical body, firming the feet, ankles and thighs. It unlocks the sacrum bone, relieving sciatica, hip and back pain (preventing and relieving arthritis), and opens out the chest. It stimulates the energies in the sacral centre, *svadhisthana* chakra, at the level of the sacrum. This centre is connected with our sexuality and security. So working in this pose is a very safe way to free the blocked energies, helping us to let go of our worries over sex and our insecurity. It brings trust in God, allowing us to go with the flow of life.

thigh parallel to the ground.) Then take the elbow onto the thigh, or the hand to the foot or ground. Go as far as you can, without collapsing the left side forwards towards the ground. Rest the left hand on the left hip and turn from deep in the right hip, turning the belly up to the left, turning the left hip to the ceiling or the sky, stretching the left leg a little more away to the outside of the left foot (see photo above). Inhale, stretch the left arm up to the ceiling, exhale, take the arm over the left ear and turn to look up under the arm (main photo, opposite). Stay there for as long as

Vrksasana (Tree Pose)

A tree has its roots firmly embedded in the earth; and the roots reach and stretch down into the ground as the branches reach up and out towards the sunlight. So in this posture we too become as the tree, firmly grounded in matter and yet at the same time lifting and opening to the light for our sustenance. If we can tune into the being of a tree it gives a oneness with trees and with mother earth.

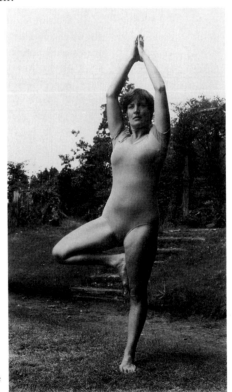

Starting in *tadasana*, feel that you are quite steady and balanced on both feet. It helps if you fix your gaze on a point ahead. A distant tree would be best, it would help you to feel the essence of a tree.

Pick up the right foot with the right hand and place it as high as possible against the left thigh, toes pointing downwards, turning the right knee out, so that the inner right thigh stretches. This will move the hip. Make sure that the left hip does not bulge out to the left, for this will take the posture out of alignment. Tuck the left hip in, stretching down from the outer hip to the outside of the foot. Lift up on the left instep all the way up the inner leg (see photo opposite).

Bring the hands together in *namaste*, the prayer position, the Indian gesture of respect, over the heart centre (as shown in the photo). Hold for at least one minute, lifting the heart up to the hands so that the whole rib-cage lifts up and opens, away from the hips. When and if you are steady, inhale; as you exhale take the arms over the head, bringing the elbows back so that the chest opens (main photo, opposite page). Do not hunch the shoulders.

Inhale while separating the hands and stretch them up towards the ceiling, exhale bringing the arms down by your side, and bring the right leg down. Repeat with the left leg. Come back to *tadasana*.

POINTS TO WATCH AND WORK ON

1. Do not take your arms over your head if you have high blood pressure or are pregnant. If the position with raised arms makes you at all dizzy or uncomfortable, keep the hands over the heart.

2. If the foot tends to slide down the standing leg, you need to stretch the outside of the foot back towards the back of the inner thigh and firmly into the standing leg. It is much easier with bare legs.

3. If you are unsteady, place one hand on the wall or chair so that you can balance.

EFFECTS

This posture brings poise, steadiness, calmness and equanimity in all circumstances of life. As well as loosening the hip-joint and

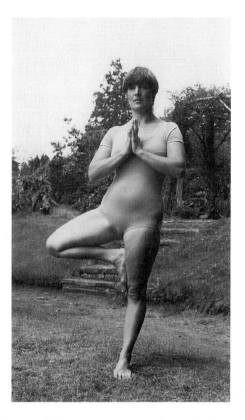

shoulders, it lifts the heart and strengthens the legs and ankles. It gives a general lifting and expansion of the energy up from the ground.

Virabhadrasana I (First Warrior Pose)

The Warrior poses embody and encourage all the attributes of the warrior in life—that of determination, strength, courage, steadfastness, and strength of the Inner Self; while softening the outer body so that it is in a relaxed receptive state. In Indian legend, Virabhadra was a mighty and powerful warrior-hero under the control of Shiva.

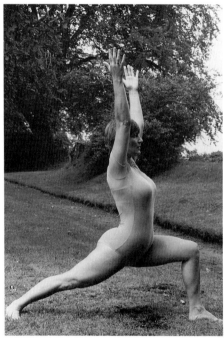

From *tadasana* take or jump the feet four to four-and-a-half feet apart and parallel to one another. Stretch firmly down the outer legs to the outside of the feet, lifting from the instep, all the way up the inner legs.

Inhale and stretch the arms to the side; exhale, taking the arms over the head, stretching up to the finger-tips without hunching the shoulders.

Turn the right foot out to the right, the left foot in 45° or more (further than for the Triangle and Stretched-flank poses). Turn the whole body from the hips right round over the right leg.

Stretch up from the heart as you inhale. On the exhalation bend the right knee so that the shin comes vertical, with the knee directly above the ankle (see photo on opposite page). Hold as long as you can, feeling the lightness and lift of the heart; and then inhale, and exhale as you come up. Bring the feet to the front and then repeat on the left side. Come back to *tadasana*.

POINTS TO WATCH AND WORK ON

1. If you have any problems such as disc lesions in your back, or your blood pressure tends to be high, or if you are pregnant, do not take your arms over your head but place your hands on your hips. This posture is a very dynamic one so do not strain in it. Work more from the heart to spread the ribs and chest, while relaxing the head, and then it will not be tiring.

2. If the back heel tends to come up, place the heel against the wall, so that the corresponding hip can move around more over the bent knee.

3. If the lower back feels strained and curved forward, stretch the whole trunk forward from the base of the spine (photo, this page). Even place the hands on the back of the chair if this helps to take the strain off the back.

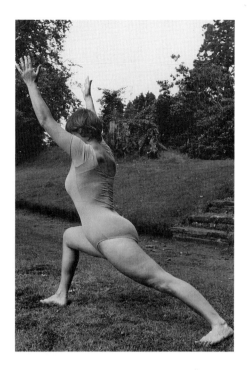

EFFECTS

This posture strengthens the legs, knees and ankles, lightens the heart, develops the chest and helps breathing; it relieves sciatica and arthritic hips; it brings out the qualities of the Inner Self that are symbolically attributed to the warrior, as mentioned in the introduction. It frees and stimulates the navel centre, *manipuraka*—the centre of our inner power—enabling us to be strong in ourselves in a safe, loving, wise way. We are able to maintain the balance of wisdom, love and power whilst being effective in our lives and in our interaction with others.

Virabhadrasana II (Second Warrior Pose)

The second Warrior pose requires skilful thought and detailed action as well as the attributes of the first Warrior pose, and is the next stage in developing the attributes of the warrior. The warrior is one who skilfully, steadfastly and calmly stands erect upon the battlefield of life, balancing himself against all opposition, inner and outer.

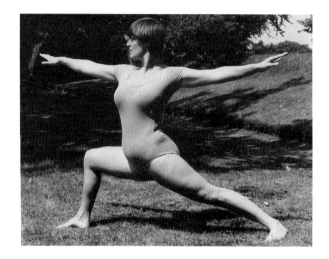

From *tadasana* take or jump the feet four to four-and-a-half feet apart, stretching the arms to the side, to shoulder level. Turn the right foot out, the left just a little in, as for *trikonasana*.

Inhale as you lift the chest, spreading the shoulders and arms a little more, exhale while bending the right knee, bringing the knee above the ankle, and keeping the right shin vertical.

Keep the weight evenly balanced between the two feet and drop the base of the spine right down evenly between the feet while stretching the rest of the spine up to the crown of the head. Stretch the left arm back to the finger-tips so that the spine is upright and the chest and ribs are spreading; look to the right finger-tips.

Take a breath and then exhale to come up. Turn the feet forwards; and then repeat on the other side. Come back to *tadasana*.

POINTS TO WATCH AND WORK ON

1. This posture requires and gives more flexibility in the hips than the first Warrior pose. If this movement of the hip does not come very easily, the back may feel strained and constricted, so

practise the posture with the back flat against the wall for a while so that the back can relax; then there will be more movement in the hip.

2. You are aiming for the right thigh to make a right angle with the right shin, when the right knee is bent. This means dropping the right buttock-bone right down and having the feet wide enough apart so that the knee does not come over the foot at all, as this strains the knee. If it is difficult to get this far down, put the left foot (this will be the back foot) against the wall, as it helps the straight leg to work better and encourages hip movement so that the full stretch of the posture comes more easily.

EFFECTS

This posture brings the effects of the first Warrior pose, as well as opening out the chest; it relieves strain in the shoulders and upper back, brings flexibility to the hips and lower back muscles and tones the abdominal organs. It also stimulates the solar plexus, the *manipuraka*, a centre of power. Power is a difficult word for some of us, particularly the British, who believe it entails being rather forceful. This of course need not and should not be the case, yet we need to be effective and strong in ourselves and in what we do. The Warrior poses bring a balance of strength and power with love and wisdom in a grounded, controlled way.

Parsvottanasana

The way the heart leads in this posture brings openness and a lightness to the chest and heart and so lifts the consciousness. Standing and walking become easier as you carry the body from the heart, instead of straining to lift it from the head and shoulders.

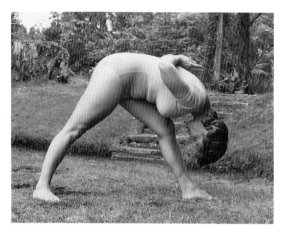

Stand in *tadasana*. Inhale, stretching the arms out to the side. As you exhale take the hands behind your back and turn your palms to place them together in *namaste*, the prayer position, turning the fingers upwards (opposite, top left). Draw the shoulders and elbows back so that the whole palm and heel of the hand come together and the fingers can stretch up towards the ceiling. Do not push the rib-cage forward but spread the back ribs against the little fingers and outside of the hands.

Then, taking the feet three to four feet apart, turn the right foot out 90° and turn the left foot in about 60° (that is, 30° to the right foot), turning the trunk right round over the right leg. Stretch the left leg firmly back, particularly the front thigh muscles, to help the left hip turn to the right (photo, lower left).

Then, inhaling, lift the heart, opening across the chest, and take the head and shoulders back; exhale as you bend forward from the hips, with the back flat and the heart leading (see main photo, above). Relax the head and neck down to place the forehead on the shin, the chest on the knee. Try to keep the elbows and shoulders back like wings. If this movement is difficult or a strain, just keep the spine extending forwards parallel to the ground, until after practice it can comfortably extend down over the leg. Inhale, and stretch forward, flattening the back to come up, exhaling to come right up. Turn to the left and repeat.

Come back to *tadasana* and gently relax the hands down, just allowing them to hang down by your sides until they feel normal. Do not shake them, as this is disturbing to the whole body.

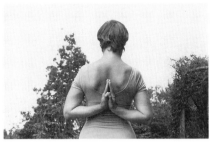

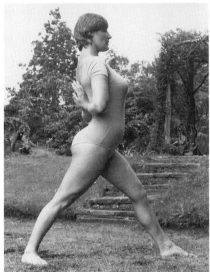

3. Always try to move from the hips evenly forward and down over the legs, with the right and left sides of the waist evenly stretched, so that you do not close up the hip of the forward leg as this will take the body out of alignment. The hips will move if you really extend and stretch the legs, lifting the insteps and the ankle-bones up away from the ground.

4. If the back heel lifts, take the heel against the wall.

EFFECTS

This posture corrects and frees round and stiff shoulders, and helps the breath to come more deeply, from the lower ribs; it increases flexibility in the hips, spine and legs, tones the abdominal organs, and loosens stiff wrists and finger-joints. Inwardly, the pose gently opens the centres from the heart upwards. The standing poses which follow work on the higher centres and are more difficult to practise, so do not be in a hurry to go on to them. Instead, work longer on this one to allow the higher centres to be gently and gradually stimulated and unblocked, which will bing a lightness of heart; and so prepare yourself for the next section of standing poses.

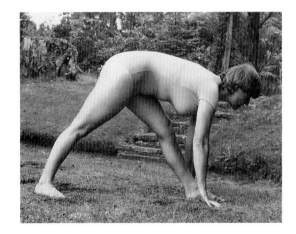

POINTS TO WATCH AND WORK ON

1. An alternative version is to keep the arms relaxed and take the hands to the ground (photo, bottom right). This is helpful when you are just starting on this posture.

2. After a while, attempt to take the hands together in *namaste* even if this is difficult; it will gradually become possible. If at first it feels impossible when practising the full posture, clasp your elbows behind your back as you bend forward in the pose.

Prasarita Padottanasana (Wide Leg-stretch Forward Bend)

Prasarita means 'expanded', 'spread' and 'extended'. This posture gives the whole body and in particular the chest and hips the feeling of being opened and released. A stable position is created in the archway of the legs from which the spine stretches up and out and then forwards and downwards. This strong and steady posture gives to the body the awareness of being the temple of the spirit.

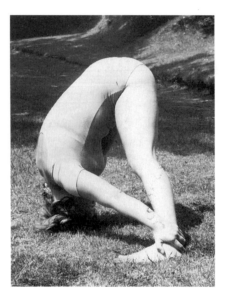

From *tadasana* take the feet four to five feet apart. With the feet parallel, hands on hips, stretch firmly down from the outer hips to the outside of the feet. Stretch up the inner legs from the lift of the insteps, as though you are making an arch of the legs.

As you inhale, stretch up away from the tops of the thighs, lifting the heart and chest. On the exhalation bend forward from the tops of the thighs and take the hands down onto the ground underneath the shoulders. Stretch forward from the tops of the thighs to the arm-pits, but keeping the hips in line with the feet, the chest moving forward and opening out to the sides, shoulders relaxed back towards the hips (illustrated top left, opposite page).

This is as far as you should go when first practising the posture, but when you feel comfortable and ready to go further, on an exhalation take the hands back in line with the feet and bring the head down towards the ground (centre, opposite page), keeping the extension of the spine and lifting the buttock-bones

— 80 —

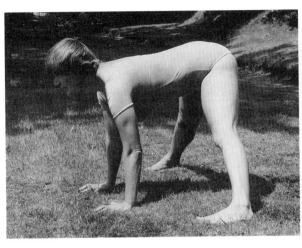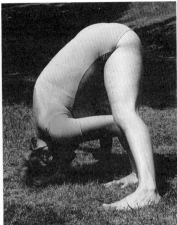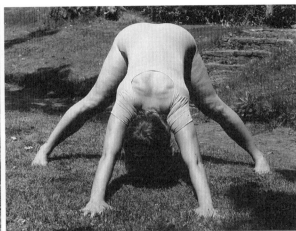

towards the ceiling.

If you are steady, take hold of the ankles to bring the upper back further down and open the chest more (main photo).

Come up out of the posture as you went into it, inhaling to stretch forward, exhaling to come right up. Come back to *tadasana*.

POINTS TO WATCH AND WORK ON

1. If you have any problem in the lower back or feel any constriction around the abdomen take your hands onto the seat of a chair and stretch forward. After practising this way for a while you will be able to go down comfortably. This position is very helpful if you are pregnant.

2. If you can get your head easily to the ground, bring your feet a little closer together so that the spine stretches more and then eventually stretches straight down, in line with the legs.

3. An extension of this posture is to take the hands as far forward as you can (keeping the hips in line with the heels) to give a Dog-pose feeling, and thus greater movement in the upper back (right-hand photo).

EFFECTS

This posture increases the blood flow to the trunk, head, legs and hips, and aids digestion. It is an alternative to the Head-stand, giving some of its effects, if that pose cannot be performed. As with *uttanasana*, this posture is practised at the end of a sequence of standing postures because it stimulates the crown centre, *sahasrara* chakra. During the sequence the energies will gradually have been freed and lifted from the base of the spine upwards, so taking the crown down onto the ground in this pose allows these stimulated energies to flow gently and freely up and down the spine, unblocking any remaining area of tightness or 'holding on' and then balancing the energies so that they meet in the heart.

Ardha Chandrasana (Half Moon Pose)

The lightness, the opening and extension in this posture gives the quality of calm serenity that can be seen and felt from the moon. The steady and quiet light of the moon will reflect itself across the chest and dance within the heart, as it slowly opens from practice of this posture.

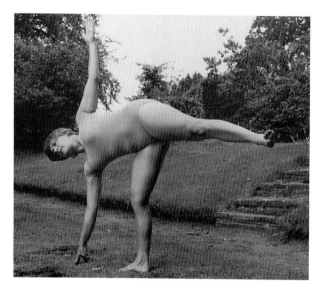

It is necessary before going on to this more difficult balancing posture, to be able to take your hand to the ground in *trikonasana*, the Triangle pose.

From *tadasana*, follow the instructions into *trikonasana*, taking your hand right down to the ground.

Once you are steady in *trikonasana*, rest the left hand down onto the hip, look to the front (not down or you will wobble); bend the right knee, take the right hand about one foot ahead of the right foot on the ground (all shown in the photo opposite,

left). On an exhalation, lift the left leg into the air in line with the hip, straightening the right leg. Keep the left leg stretched (photo opposite, right). When and if you are steady, straighten the left arm up towards the ceiling, spreading the ribs, opening the chest forwards and lifting the left hip to the ceiling (illustrated above). Hold the pose as long as you feel steady.

To come down, bend the right knee, keeping the left leg firm, and stretch it back and down to the ground so that you come back into the Triangle pose, then inhale, and exhale to come up.

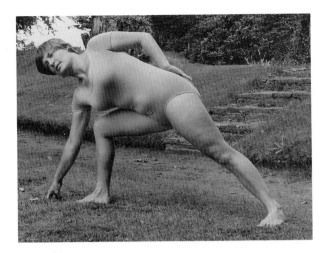 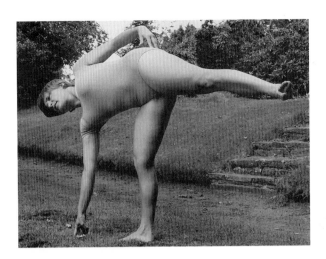

Repeat on the left side. Then come back to *tadasana*.

POINTS TO WATCH AND WORK ON

1. If you feel unsteady in this posture, which is usual when first starting to practise it, or if it feels a strain on the hip and the standing leg, then practise the posture with the back flat against the wall, so that the left heel stretches up against the wall when going to the right, and vice versa.

2. If it is difficult to take the hand to the ground, then use a chair or block to put the hand on, so that you do not have to go so far when first practising. You should have practised *trikonasana*

for several months or even a year in order to have the steadiness and balance for this posture.

EFFECTS

This posture brings mobility and lightness to the hips and legs, increasing the circulation in these areas, while freeing the chest and upper back and loosening the shoulders. Inwardly it opens the heart centre, the *anahata* chakra, softening the heart and therefore softening our approach and attitudes to those close to us—releasing any 'hard-heartedness' we may have acquired by blocking the heart centre, so that we are free to love without fear.

Virabhadrasana III (Third Warrior Pose)

As well as sharing the attributes of the first and second poses, the third Warrior pose goes on to develop poise, stamina and endurance in its fine balance of the energies throughout the body, especially in the legs, arms and hips. Practise Warrior I and Warrior II for some months before going on to this one.

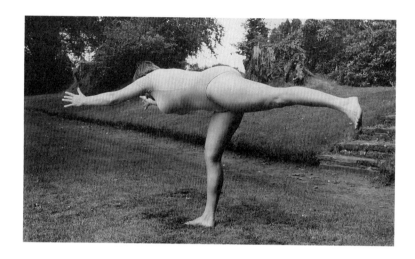

Follow the instructions into *virabhadrasana I* (photo opposite, upper picture), stretch up a little more on an inhalation, and as you exhale stretch the trunk down over the right thigh (opposite, below). Inhale as you bring the weight forward more over the right foot; exhale, stretch the right leg straight, lifting the left leg to hip height; and extend the trunk, arms and head forwards, keeping the hips in line (main photo, above). Do not hold this pose for long at first, and if you are very unsteady put your hands on a chair. When you are familiar with the posture, either with the chair or without, stretch up from the right heel into the right

hip, turning the belly from the left hip into the right hip to open out the latter. Then extend the left heel back to stretch the thigh away from the left hip, at the same time extending forwards to the finger-tips. The whole body is now extending and lengthening into the pose. Keep that extension as you come down so that the left leg stretches back and away out of the left hip and the trunk extends up, to bring you back into the first Warrior pose, and exhale to come up.

Repeat, turning to the left side. Relax down into *uttanasana* after finishing this posture.

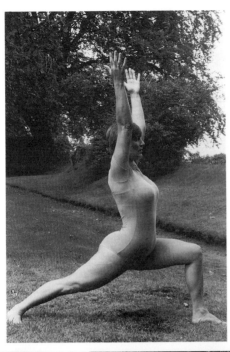

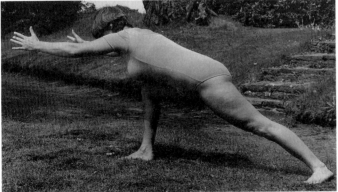

POINTS TO WATCH AND WORK ON

1. It is a good idea to use a chair or ledge at first or if the pose feels too much for you, as it helps the movement in the hips, which is where the whole pose comes from. You can then make sure that the hips are parallel—so watch the tendency to lift the hip of the lifted leg above that of the standing leg: they need to be level, then the spine stretches straight out of the sacrum.

2. Watch that you do not over-extend the standing leg by jamming the knee back. Have this knee a little bent when first practising this pose if you need to, because then you will have more control from the hips. Then stretch up into the buttock-bone of the standing leg from the stretch down of the heel, so that the leg will eventually straighten without locking.

EFFECTS

This posture gives poise and balance in standing because it brings the weight down more through the balls of the feet. We often stand very heavily on the heels, which tends to make the mind and body very sluggish and heavy and as though we are lacking in energy. Making the balance more evenly centred lightens the whole body and mind, giving vitality and joy.

The pose also tones and strengthens all the abdominal organs, giving vibrant health.

The stretch forwards on the spine opens the thymus gland, situated just under the breast-bone. This gland controls the energy in our body. Until recently it was thought that it atrophied in childhood but it has now been discovered that it only stops working just a moment before death. It in fact plays a very important part in the amount of energy we have in our system, so this pose is very energizing and stimulating.

Parivrtta Trikonasana (Reverse Triangle Pose)

In postures which stretch the spine straight, it is said that the lessons of living on the earth are being learnt; but as the spine becomes more extended it gradually twists and turns itself heavenwards, like the spirit winging homeward toward heaven, to learn the lessons of heaven. The increased flexibility that the Reverse Triangle pose gives to the spine extends the consciousness and opens the heart to fly upwards.

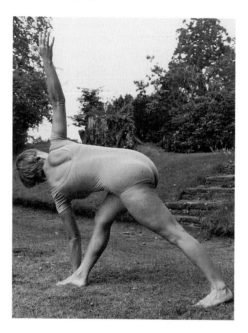

From *tadasana* take the feet three to four feet apart stretching the arms to the side as you inhale; exhale and turn the left foot in to the right 45°, turning the knee as well to face to the right, and the right foot out to the right 90°, keeping the right heel in line with the left instep.

Inhaling, stretch the trunk up off the thighs, stretching the feet firmly down into the ground; exhaling, turn the trunk from the very base of the spine right around over the right foot (see photo opposite).

As you exhale, take the right hand onto the right hip, stretch the left arm right out over the right leg and down to the right foot, or to the ground if you can, without caving the chest in. Turn the whole trunk to face towards the opposite way from which you have been facing, stretch the right side of the rib cage up towards the ceiling, the left side towards the ground so that the whole trunk can stretch out, extending the crown of the head forwards, the base of the spine back away from you.

When and if you are steady, stretch the right arm up towards the ceiling (main photo, opposite page). Turn the head to look up to the right finger-tips.

Inhale to come up, exhale and turn to repeat on the left side. Then come back to *tadasana*.

POINTS TO WATCH AND WORK ON

1. In this posture the spine should eventually be stretched straight out to the side, as for the Triangle pose, but there is a tendency to round the back when first starting to practise. If you feel that your spine is not stretching as much as it could, then put the left hand on a block or chair when moving to the right (and vice versa) so that you do not hunch up in your attempt to get the hand down onto the ground, as that destroys the aim of the posture.

2. If the back heel comes off the ground as you go into the pose, then the hip of that leg will close up. To prevent this and increase the stretch in the back leg, place the heel (*only* the heel) against the wall so that you can stretch it back into the wall. This also helps the spine stretch out and forward.

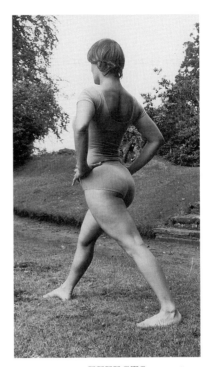

EFFECTS

This posture increases the flexibility of the hips and spine, tones up the kidneys, liver and abdominal organs, works the adrenal glands and opens the rib-cage, chest and heart. It works to free the energy in the throat centre, the *visuddha* chakra, the trust centre, so enabling us to trust the process of life and trust those around us.

Parivrtta Parsvakonasana (Reverse Stretched-flank Pose)

As with *parivrtta trikonasana*, this pose moves out of the more earthy direction of *utthita parsvakonasana* to revolve up heavenwards. It is an intense extension together with an intense twist so as to give a deep spiralling movement of the energy from the sacrum to the brow. Do not practise it, therefore, until you have spent a good long while on the simpler standing postures.

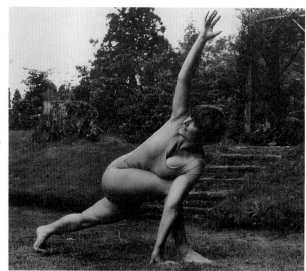

Inhale, spread the legs wide apart (about five feet), and extend the arms to the side while exhaling. Turn the right leg and foot 90° to the right, the left toes a little to the right; exhale, bend the right knee to come into the second Warrior pose. Take your hands onto your hips, then turn the whole trunk over the right thigh (photo: opposite page, top left); as you stretch forward, stretch the left arm down against the outside of the right foot, levering the arm against the knee to turn the ribs and shoulders, and thus the chest towards the sky or ceiling, resting the right hand on the right hip. In the initial stages you may need to take the left arm down to the left side of the right leg, but still working to get the turn in the trunk of the body (opposite, top right). It is very likely, especially in the first years of practice, that the left heel will need to lift and turn upwards, as in the photo, in order to turn from the left hip. On an exhalation, extend the right arm over the right ear (main photo, above). If you feel that this closes up the chest, then keep the hand down on the hip. Hold for as long as the body will extend into it. To come up, inhale, return to the second Warrior pose; exhale, come right up and repeat to the left. Then return to *tadasana* and relax down into *uttanasana*.

POINTS TO WATCH AND WORK ON

1. If the turn of the trunk feels very difficult, practise initially with your back against a wall, so that when you turn you will be able to place both hands on the wall and stretch them into it to lever the chest around (photo: below right, opposite page). Just go this far until the turn feels easier; doing this greatly increases the amount of turn, so do not be in a hurry to go further.

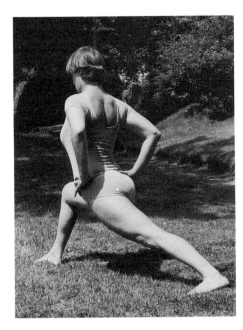

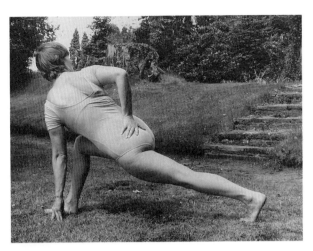

the *ajna* chakra—the centre that relates to the planet as a whole. Thus we do it to help us to feel oneness with the earth and mankind at an inner level; even to feel the feelings of the earth, the animal kingdom, the plant kingdom, the mineral kingdom. It gives that sense of us *all* experiencing what we *each* experience.

2. If it feels difficult to extend the back leg with the heel lifted, place the heel so that it touches and so can stretch into the wall. This will improve the work and extension in the back leg, so the thigh will not so readily collapse towards the ground.

3. If the chest feels as if it closes in, do not go so far down into the posture, but stretch up and out more. Just take the left elbow against the right knee, or use blocks to place the hand on, rather than taking it right down to the ground.

EFFECTS

This posture helps elimination and so cleanses and purifies the whole system, stimulating the circulation of blood around the spine and abdominal organs, and thus revitalizes and energizes the whole system, strengthening the legs and spine, extending all the muscles and ligaments. This is because it frees the energy in

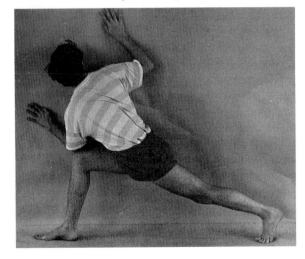

Uttanasana (Standing Forward Bend)

This posture rests and relaxes the body between the other standing postures, by extending the spine from the base to the crown of the head, and down towards the feet, allowing the consciousness to extend from the lower self to the Higher Self. The more the spine extends and stretches, the more the Higher Self awakens, as the subtle energies that run down the spine are aligned and awakened, so releasing the higher consciousness.

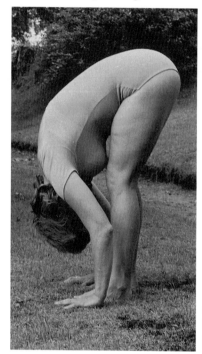

Stand in *tadasana* with the feet hip-width apart, inhale and stretch up away from the tops of the thighs lifting the heart. It can be helpful to place the fingers just between the top front thighs and hips to make space there and feel that you will be bending from there. Exhale and bend forward from the top of the thighs, keeping the back flat as you go down, taking the finger-tips to the ground underneath the shoulders (photo: opposite, above right).

Then walk the hands back towards the feet, relaxing the whole of the upper body down, with the crown of the head moving towards the ground, so that the neck stretches and relaxes, rib-cage spreading, breathing evenly (main photo, above). But keep the legs stretching up from the heels to the buttock-bones, and from the insteps all the way up the inner legs.

The spine will stretch a little more, if you take hold of the arms at the elbows, as shown (photo: lower right). Stay there until you

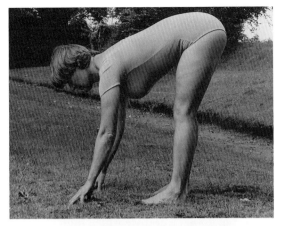

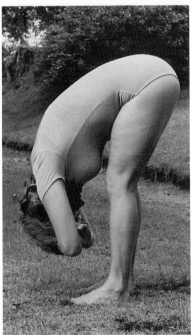

feel rested, refreshed and extended in the spine. To come out of the posture inhale, walk the hands forward, lift the head, stretch the chest forwards, and exhaling come right up to standing with the back flat, the shoulders opening out and back.

POINTS TO WATCH AND WORK ON

1. If you have lower back problems in the lumbar region, sciatica, or uneven hips, do not bend right down but stretch forward onto a chair, so that the spine extends and evens out. This version is also helpful when you are pregnant.

2. If you feel dizzy or heavy in the head, do not go right down but use the chair.

3. Do not over-extend the backs of the knees so the knee-caps are jammed into the knees, as this creates a counter-balancing curvature in the lumbar spine. Go into the posture with the knees slightly bent as shown and feel how the spine can extend and lengthen much more. Then extend the heels down into the ground, the buttock-bones up to the ceiling so that the whole of the backs of the legs stretch and extend, not just the knees. Then let the knees bend as you come up. It is very damaging to the lower spine and sacrum to go in and out of this posture with the knees locked back.

EFFECTS

The awakening of the higher consciousness in this posture relieves depression and heaviness in the mind if the posture is held for two or more minutes. It tones the liver, spleen, kidneys, and stomach; and relieves pain and strain during menstruation. Spinal nerves are rejuvenated and the heart beats are slowed down so that one feels relaxed, refreshed, calm and peaceful after coming up out of the *asana*. It allows the subtle energies to move freely up from the base of the spine and down from the crown of the head, freeing the energy in the crown centre, so making us more aware of our connection to the Universe and our oneness with all life.

CHAPTER SIX

Forward-Bending Postures

The answer to your own individual problem and heartache is to surrender all to God. Be still within, be calm. Do not try to overdrive your life. Be calm, do your work quietly; live as the flowers live, opening your heart to the sunlight of God's love.

White Eagle, THE QUIET MIND

Postures which take the spine forward surrender the ego to the Higher Self. This is the effect of letting the head come forward towards the feet. Bowing to or washing someone's feet has always been a gesture of humility in the East. In India the *chela* (pupil) touches the feet of the *guru* as a sign of respect and acknowledgment; in the Bible there is the beautiful story of Mary Magdalene anointing the feet of Jesus, a gesture which indicates that He is her Master. So the head coming towards the feet has the inner effect of the ego gradually letting go its hold, thus allowing the Higher or Inner Self to shine through the outer self and bringing calmness and serenity.

AWARENESS AND ATTENTION

In each of the forward-bending poses, be aware of letting go the mind in the head. Let go the control it has on the rest of the body, let go its desire to lead, to force and to strain. Let the forward movement always come from the base of the spine and travel along the whole spine as you move, so that the head follows the rest of the body. Practising in this way you will let go of the ego's strong hold on the body as a whole and move instead from the mind in the heart, so that you bring humility and gentleness to the action.

Dandasana (Staff Pose)

Danda, the staff, is the symbol of authority, of someone in control. This posture brings control of the spine. When the spine can be moved and extended by the will then the whole body, and therefore the whole of your life, comes under the control of the Inner Self.

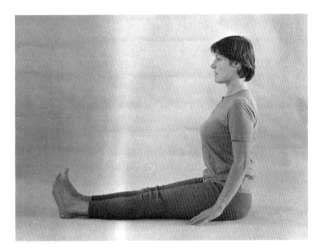

Sit on the floor with your legs stretched straight out in front of you and the feet hip-width apart. Take hold of the buttock-bones with your hands and move them back away from the heels so that you can feel an even extension from the one to the other. Stretch the spine upwards, lifting the heart, spreading the chest and ribs to the side (illustrated above). It can help to have the finger-tips just on the ground, wherever they can be of most assistance in stretching the spine up without hunching the shoulders.

If you feel that you are leaning backwards, have the hands a little behind the hips so that you can stretch forward and up a little more. If you feel that you hunch forward, have the hands level with the thighs and feel as though you are stretching the finger-tips back along the ground toward your hips: this lifts the front of the body. Breathe normally throughout this posture and only hold it as long as you feel that you can stretch up into it. Although it is a simple posture, if you are used to supporting your back against a chair it will be hard work for the back muscles at first, but the posture will gradually strengthen them and it will become easier to hold.

POINTS TO WATCH AND WORK ON

1. Do not worry if the backs of the legs ache: this is just because they are not used to stretching evenly. If you have practised

any kind of sport and then stopped, the muscles are particularly likely to have tightened. The ache will go in time and is what is described in the introduction as good pain! The stretch of the hamstring muscles will enable the spine to stretch up.

2. If the pelvis and lower spine curve back and it feels impossible to stretch up from the base of the spine, sit on a folded blanket or block. This will rotate the pelvis forwards and enable you to stretch up more.

EFFECTS

This posture extends the hamstring muscles down the backs of the legs, strengthens the back muscles, and tones up the lower abdominal organs. It brings strength, stretch and control to the spine and so to the whole central nervous system. Thus it creates stillness of mind and body.

Parvatasana (Cross-legged Forward Bend)

This is a rather easier variation of the classic *parvatasana*, which is traditionally practised in the Lotus pose, *padmasana*. It helps very much in working towards the Lotus pose. It also frees the hip-joints, which is necessary for taking the spine forward, and so can also be practised as part of the seated posture sequence.

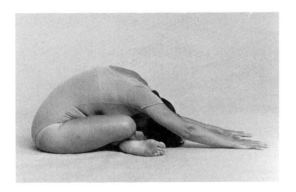

From *dandasana*, cross the legs, the left leg in first and then the right. Do not have the feet tucked right up under you: bring them out so that they are under the knees, the shins parallel to the hips, making a squarish shape (photo overleaf, top left). Keep the heels stretched, as this works to free the hips. Turn over the right knee, taking your hands either side of the knee. Inhale, lengthen the spine up, and exhaling stretch forward over the right leg (opposite page, lower left). Relax there for one or two minutes, letting the left buttock-bone relax back to the ground, if it tends to lift. To come up, inhale, lifting your head and chest; exhale, and straighten the spine up. Turn over to the left leg and repeat. Then come to the front, take the hands forward over the legs, spine straight, chest forward and up.

That may be as far as you can go when first practising this pos-

ture. To go further, stretch the spine forward and lift the chest up as you inhale; relax forward and down towards the ground as you exhale (main photo, above). Relax there by taking your awareness, with the breath, into the hip-joints and legs as you inhale; as you exhale, relax the whole upper body forward and down a little more. On the next inhalation, spread and soften the belly down into the hips and sacrum. Then repeat the whole posture with the legs crossed the other way round.

POINTS TO WATCH AND WORK ON

1. The reaction or 'good pain' felt in the hips and outer thighs in this posture is very beneficial in freeing the hips. The feeling of

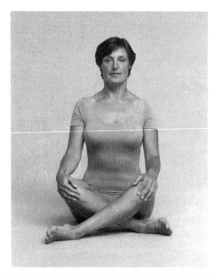

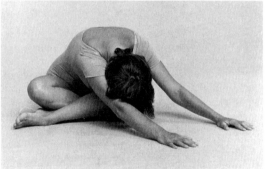

pain needs to be relaxed into and worked through in order to move the hip-joint, so just take your awareness there and 'let go' into it.

2. It is very helpful to use a block or chair to relax forward onto. The effect of relaxing the head onto something firm is a release of the hip-joint, as the outer mind will then let go to allow this to happen. If the hips and lower back are very stiff, or if you are pregnant, you will need to use a chair as you move to each side, as well as forward.

EFFECTS

This posture increases the blood supply and the mobility of the hips, and frees the lumbar spine out of the hips. It relieves sciatica, lower back problems, stiffness and arthritis in the hips, and tones the abdominal organs, so it is of use in any problems of the intestines and reproductive organs. The effect of taking the head forward and down, resting the brow on the floor or a chair or block, is to quieten the busy outer mind. This in turn produces a 'letting go' in the sacrum and coccyx and the energy is able to move freely up and down the spine.

Janu Sirsasana (Forward Bend over each Leg)

Janu means 'knee' and *sirsa* means 'head'; but *janu* also means 'soul', so that in this posture, by bringing the head to the knee you are also surrendering the head-mind to the soul-mind, you are creating the still lake, so that the soul can be clearly reflected in the outer self and outer life.

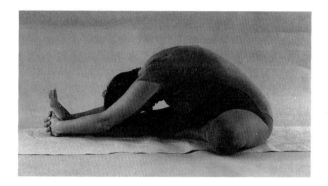

Sit in *dandasana*; bend the left knee up towards you and out to the left, placing the left foot alongside the right thigh so that the heel is between the groins of the two thighs, the top of the foot on the ground.

Turn your whole trunk right round over the right leg, stretching the left knee and thigh away and out to the left; take the left arm to the other side of the right leg, the right hand onto the ground behind you (first photo overleaf).

Inhale, stretch the spine upwards. Exhale, twist the spine to the right, levering the left hand against the right leg, the right finger-tips stretching into the ground to lift and open the chest and spiral the spine to the right. Stay there as long as you are stretching up into it. Come out on an exhalation. Repeat on the other side. Return to *dandasana*. Twisting the spine first of all helps you to go forwards in the forward bend.

Now again bend the left knee, but this time as you take it out to

the side take it back behind the level of the hip on the ground so that the left heel is at the root of the left thigh.

Turn out of the left hip to face over the right leg. Inhale, stretch the spine up, take both hands either side of the right leg; exhale and go forwards, keeping the stretch of the spine and the openness of the chest so that the chest is going forward towards the right foot. Take the hands down either side of the right leg, and then take hold of the right foot (top picture, overleaf, right) or have a belt around the foot to help the upward stretch of the spine (lower picture). Turn the belly out of the left hip to the right, turn the ribs from the left, opening out the right side of the rib-cage as you go forwards.

When the belly and ribs can relax down on the straight leg, then let the head relax to the shin (main photo, this page).

Do not take the head down too soon as this will curve the spine, but stay in the position of the first photo and then the second for

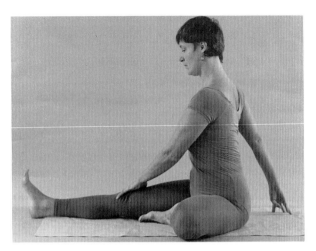

the first few months of practising the posture, if your spine needs to stretch first.

Inhale to lift your head and exhale to come up. Repeat on the other side.

POINTS TO WATCH AND WORK ON

1. If you feel at all constricted around the abdomen, if the back hunches up or if it feels difficult to turn over the straightened leg, then stay in the position of the photo above, with the back straight. By practising this position for a while without trying to strain and pull yourself forward, you will later be able to go right forward without any trouble. If it is difficult to reach your feet, use a belt around the ball of your foot as suggested.

2. If the bent knee is painful and does not relax to the ground, put some support underneath it—a folded blanket, book or block—so that it can relax.

3. If the bent knee does relax down to the ground, gradually try to take it further back behind the hips to give more mobility and stretch in the hips and thighs.

EFFECTS

This posture tones up the liver and kidneys and regulates the adrenals, so aiding digestion. It relieves sciatica and stiffness in the hips and legs. It quietens and stills the mind.

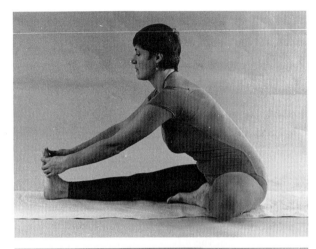

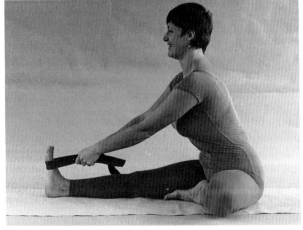

Ardha Baddha Padma Paschimottanasana
(Half Lotus Forward Bend)

Janu sirsasana and *parvatasana* need to be practised for some while until the body is ready to go on to this pose, because it needs much releasing in the hip-joint, and also in the sacrum.

The lotus flower has its roots embedded in the mud at the bottom of the pond, which represents the subconscious. The stem of the lotus reaches up through the waters of the pond—the emotions. The lotus then flowers on the surface of the water. The flowering of the lotus is thus symbolic of the awakening of consciousness—the recognition of who we really are, the realization of the divinity within us.

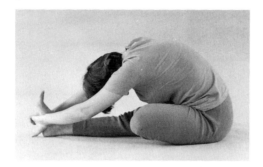

For this reason moving into the Lotus and Half Lotus poses entails release of all the held-in emotions (fear, anger, desire, resentment) in the hips, the belly and the sacrum bone. As long as they are held in the subconscious they will be there to trouble us and hold us back. Many people resist the deep movement in this pose and just move from the knee and ankle, so that the feet are collapsing down into the groin. This has been termed an 'unflowering lotus', and it creates problems in the knee-joint, indicating that a lesson of humility needs to be learned, the lesson of acceptance of all the emotions within us. Although we are not 'above them', our emotions do not need to rule us. Bringing them out, in the Lotus pose, enables us to look at them honestly and then detach ourselves from them, and so release the hold they have on us. Be sure therefore, that the movement of taking the leg into the Lotus pose comes from deep in the hip-joint so that the energy is released in the hips and can stretch up through the spine. The spine represents the stem of the lotus rising up through the waters of the emotions. The lotus in the crown chakra can then flower and so awaken the consciousness, which in this pose is then taken towards the feet in humility, understanding and acceptance of our true nature—which embraces both the inner and the outer, the higher and the lower, the divine and the human.

Sit in *dandasana*, take the left fingers behind the left knee, and hold the left heel with the right hand, lifting it up to the height of the knee. Stretch the thigh forward to bring the knee in, in line with the hip, taking the left hand onto the left calf, turning it towards the ceiling (see photo, below left). Take the left foot right up to rest on the root of the right thigh (photo below right). If this is not possible, have the foot further down the right thigh but not collapsing down into the groin. If you look at the feet of the Buddha in pictures of him seated in this pose, they are right up over the thigh with the soles of the feet and the toes all opening out like the petals of the lotus. This is what you are aiming at, and you will never achieve it if you do the posture in a lazy, easy way by letting the foot close up. It is better to practise *janu sirsasana* to get the movement in the hip before going on to this pose. When the foot is as high up as you can get it, then take hands behind you and stretch the spine up (photo opposite, top). This is a pose in itself, so if the knee is up in the air do not try going forwards at all as that will just curve and collapse the spine. Go on stretching

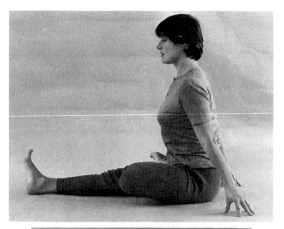

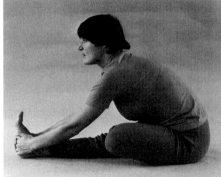

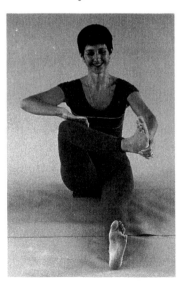

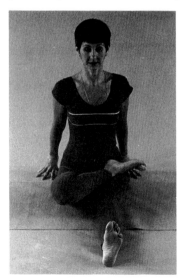

the spine straight up, taking the knee forwards and in towards the straight leg, with the heel stretching away. All these movements will work to release and move the hip-joint.

If the knee is relaxing down towards the ground, then by using your hands beside you to stretch up, lift the belly and lower back up over the foot to take the spine forwards, the head towards the foot. Bring the hands forward to take hold of the right foot. Keep the spine stretched as you go forwards (lower photo, this column). The pose in this picture is a much better one to hold than letting the spine curve and collapse backwards in order to force the head down towards the leg, which only brings in the impatient ego that wants to force and control. Only go forwards when the spine can stretch over the foot, always moving forwards on an exhalation, and stretching up on an inhalation. The further position is shown in the main photo, page 99.

To come up, inhale, stretch the spine up into *dandasana*; and exhale to stretch the leg out. Repeat on the other side.

POINTS TO WATCH AND WORK ON

1. Many people complain about the pressure of the ankle of the bent leg on the thigh of the straight leg. This pressure is good pain, and if you can relax into it, it will release a lot of the tension that we hold in the thighs. It is helped by stretching the ankle of the bent leg away more and bringing the foot more over the straight thigh. Keep the heel of the straight leg stretched and its foot stretched up. Do not let the foot flop out to the side.

EFFECTS

This pose brings flexibility and release to the hips, knees and ankle-joints. It helps rounded shoulders by opening the chest out. It brings freedom from unruly emotions, as explained in detail in the introduction, giving peace and calm to the whole system. It tones the uro-genitary system and the abdominal muscles and so is good for menopausal and period problems, and prostate and bladder problems.

Triang Mukhaikapada Paschimottanasana
(Forward Bend with one Leg in Hero Pose)

This pose has a balancing, centering effect after the last three poses, as it turns the hip and knee in the other direction. It increases flexibility in the hips, and this helps release the sacrum, knee-joint and belly.

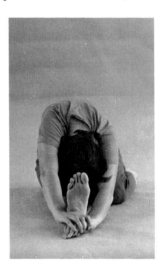

Sit in *dandasana*, the Staff pose, and take the left leg back into *virasana*, the Hero pose (left foot by left hip). Take the finger-tips into the ground, in order to stretch the spine upwards, opening the chest, straightening the back (photo: opposite page). Inhale as you stretch the spine up, and as you exhale take the fingers forward, either side of the straight thigh. Remain evenly balanced over both thighs. Do not go so far down that the spine slumps backwards.

If the balance is even on the buttocks, take the hands around the foot of the straight leg and relax forward and down, chest towards the foot (main photo, above). If you collapse over to the straight leg side, stretch the straight leg away, stretch the toes up towards the sky, and turn the heel of the bent leg more away from the hip. This will bring the spine into even balance between the two thighs. To come up, inhale, lift your head; exhale, stretch the spine up and the bent leg out; and repeat on the other side.

POINTS TO WATCH AND WORK ON

1. If you are sitting unevenly on the buttock-bones after taking

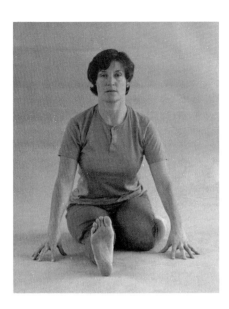

one leg back into the Hero pose, then put a block or book or firm cushion under the buttock of the straight leg.

2. If you feel curved and collapsed in the small of the back and chest, then use a belt around the feet to give an upwards stretch of the spine.

EFFECTS

In the whole series of forward bends this is an important balancing pose, giving the movement of the hip-joint with the knee bent into Hero pose.

It helps strain or sprains in the ankle, when support of a blanket may be needed under the ankle. It corrects misshapen feet, dropped arches and curled toes, and enlarged big toe-joints. It tones the abdominal organs and like the other forward bends brings calm and quiet to the head-mind, by extending the spine and head forwards.

Marichyasana I

Eventually *marichyasana I* is a forward bend, but it is better to keep stretched upright in it at first so that it is more of a twist and a preparation for *marichyasana II* and *III*. As with all the very simple twists it is very effective at stretching, strengthening and spiralling the spine around to bring to life the whole spinal column, spinal cord and corresponding nerve endings and endocrine glands.

It has been placed in the sequence of forward bends as it is one of the postures in the sequence building up to *paschimottanasana*.

If the posture is new to you practise it as a twist for the first few months or years (see Points to Watch, nos. 1 and 2).

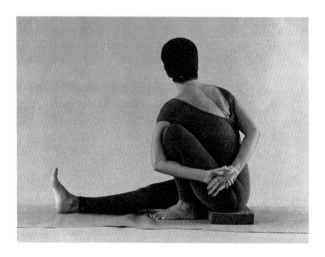

Sit in *dandasana* (Staff pose) and bend the left knee up so that the left foot is on the ground, close to the left buttock. Take the right hand onto the ground behind you, and take the left arm against the inside of the left knee, the hand stretched against the outside of the straight right leg. Stretch the spine up on an inhalation, and as you exhale spiral the spine around to the right. This is the first stage of the posture, just go this far if it is new to you

(photo: top left, opposite).

For the second stage, stretch forward over the right leg, extending the left arm forward (right-hand photo, opposite) and then take the left arm around the left leg and the right arm around your back so that the left hand takes hold of the right wrist. Stretching the spine up, twist to the right first of all; and then exhaling, turn the whole trunk to face over the right leg and

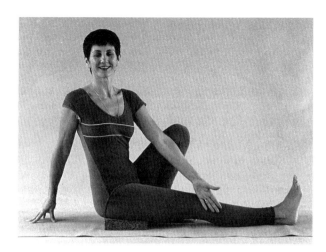

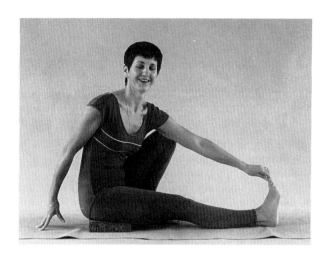

stretch forwards towards the right foot. Keep the chest open, and moving towards the foot. Stay in the pose for as long as you can stretch the chest forwards and down towards the right foot (main photo, opposite). Inhale to lift your head, exhale to come up releasing the left leg; repeat, bending up the right leg and twisting to the left.

POINTS TO WATCH AND WORK ON

1. Do not be in a hurry to go into the final stage of the pose especially if you feel closed in the chest and hunched in the shoulders. Twisting up and around is a very good release on the shoulders; so stay in the second stage until you feel you have moved your shoulders.

2. If your spine feels very curved when you take the arms around the leg, stay in the first stage, until it has lengthened; this may take several months, but that does not matter as there will be more movement in the spine.

EFFECTS

This pose has all the benefits of twisting the spine and stretching it forwards but works especially on the upper back and heart centre. By releasing the shoulders and opening the chest the dorsal spine stretches and so the heart centre opens. So it is especially helpful for those who have closed their hearts to others in protection and fear, as it gently releases the armouring, for if we open our hearts to others in love they too will open to us.

Upavistha Konasana (Seated Angle Pose)

The wide angle and firm extension of this posture gives very much the inner awareness that 'I am not only the body but beyond and above', although we remain firmly rooted and stable on the earth. It is a posture that babies often adopt when first sitting. It gives them stability as well as freedom of movement as their spines are so supple and yet firm and straight. In this posture we can begin to get back to that feeling of flexibility with steadiness in mind and body.

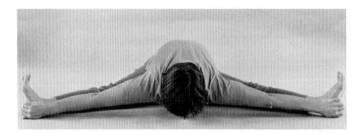

From *dandasana*, the Staff posture, take the legs as wide apart as you can, freeing the thigh-bone out of the hip-joint, extending the heels away so that the backs of the legs are stretched firmly and evenly down to the ground, from the buttock-bones to the heels (photo: top left, opposite). The more the legs extend the more the spine is able to stretch up; it can help either to take the hands behind the hips (finger-tips on the ground), or against the inside of the leg, but not so that they pull the legs up off the ground. Lift the chest by spreading the palms down into the legs. Then turn around over the right leg, feeling the turn coming from deep in the left hip, so that the sacrum on the left moves in and up, and the belly moves from the left to the right side. Take the left hand to the other side of the right leg (as shown for *janu sirsasana* in the first photo on p. 98). Lifting the chest, stretch the spine up as you inhale; as you exhale come forward over the right leg (middle photo, opposite). Relaxing the left shoulder down, turn the right ribs to the right so that the left ribs come round over the right leg,

moving the head towards the right foot, hands either side of the foot (bottom picture) or taking hold of the foot. Relax there for a few moments but keep turning from deep in the left hip, forwards along the right leg, stretching the left leg out and away to the left to open the left hip and relax the left buttock down. Inhale to come up; exhale to turn and go over the left leg, and repeat the whole posture to the left.

The next stage of the posture is to go forwards. Do this only when the spine can really stretch right forward from the base, so that the whole length of the front of the body moves forward from the pubic bone. Otherwise you will cave in at the waist, constricting the spine and internal organs. Keep the lift of the heart so that it comes forward first, and as you bend forward, spread the arms to take hold of either ankle (illustrated top right, opposite). Inhale to lift, exhale as you move forwards; only take the head down when the chest can touch the ground (main picture, this page). Inhale to come up and, exhaling, bring the legs together.

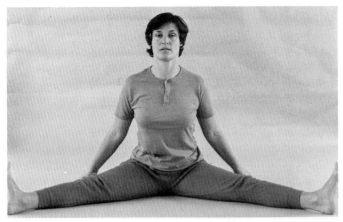

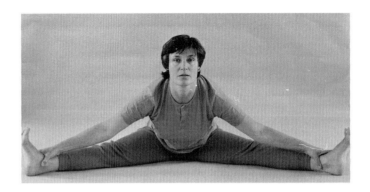

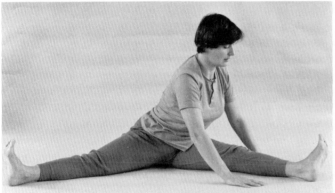

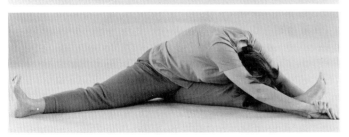

POINTS TO WATCH AND WORK ON

1. The spine stretches much more if you keep extending up, so do not go down forward over the legs too soon. If the spine curves you cannot move any more, whereas the stretch forward of the spine will eventually come with practice. Sitting on a block or folded blanket will help the spine to stretch. It is also helpful to use a belt around your foot (as in the final photo for *janu sirsasana* on p. 98).

2. If you are nearly onto the ground when bending forward, it can be a help to put a block or a few books underneath your head or ribs, in order to relax more into the posture and go a little further.

EFFECTS

This posture frees hip-joints and trapped nerves, relieves sciatica, improves the circulation in the pelvic region and is of great benefit during pregnancy and menstruation. It tones, controls and regularises the lower abdominal organs, particularly the ovaries and the prostate. It gives a feeling of openness and freedom to the whole system.

Paripurna Navasana (Boat Pose)

Paripurna means 'entire' or 'complete'. *Nava* means 'boat': this pose resembles a boat floating on the surface of the water. Although it is not strictly a forward-bending posture it follows the pattern of the forward bends.

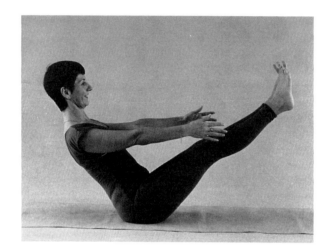

METHOD FOR BEGINNERS: from *dandasana* bend the legs up towards you and hold the backs of the thighs; inhaling, lift your chest, straightening the spine (photo top left, opposite). Exhale, stretch your legs out straight to make a right angle with your body. Breathe normally there and go on stretching and lifting the spine from the base and extending the legs through to the heels (top right).

When you feel steady and stretched and have found your point of balance, extend the arms out in front of you, palms facing each other, breathing normally (main photo, this page). Exhale to

relax down into *dandasana*; repeat, then lie down on your back.

WHEN THE BEGINNERS' METHOD HAS BEEN MASTERED: from *dandasana*, keeping the spine straight, let the whole back move backwards from the base, whilst lifting the legs from the floor (stretching the heels away) so that they maintain the right angle with the spine. Then stretch the arms forward as before with palms facing each other. Stretch up into the posture, and keep lifting and opening the chest, breathing normally, for as long as you can. Then relax back into *dandasana*, and lie down on your back.

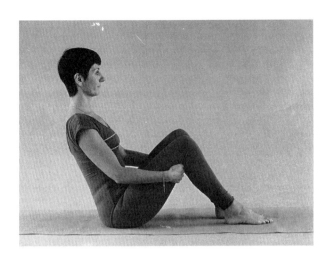 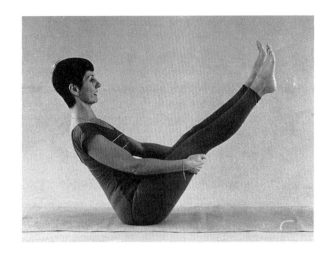

POINTS TO WATCH AND WORK ON

1. Relax the belly whilst doing *paripurna navasana*; rather, use the back muscles to stretch up into the pose.

2. Do not let the spine sink back onto the ground: use the back muscles to lift it up.

EFFECTS

Mr Iyengar says of this pose that 'it enables us to grow old gracefully and comfortably'! It does this by strengthening the lower back muscles, which tend to weaken because we always support them in chairs so that they do not do the work they are intended to do in holding the back upright. Practice of this pose will enable you to sit without spinal support and prevents the damage to the lower back which is so common among those who continually use chairs, cushions and supports. It also tones the kidneys and intestines, relieves gas and bloating in the abdomen and reduces fat around the waistline. It helps create a strong straight spine, which is in itself invigorating and uplifting to the spirits.

Paschimottanasana (Sitting Forward Bend)

All the previous variations on a forward bend work towards and help this classical forward bend, one of the main postures of yoga. Taking the head to the feet in this way is humbling and quietening, as it surrenders the ego by taking the head-mind to the feet, the understanding—'under-the-standing'—the feet signifying soul-understanding. See the introduction to the Half-lotus Forward Bend for a deeper understanding of the effect of moving the spine forward and taking the crown towards the feet.

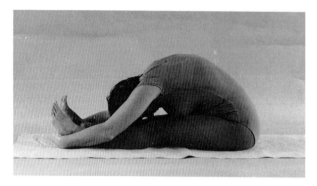

Sit in *dandasana*, the Staff pose; stretch the spine up as you inhale. As you exhale, come forward, keeping the back straight and the heart lifted (opposite, left-hand photo). Gradually take the finger-tips forward towards the feet. Use the finger-tips, stretching down and back into the ground to keep the lift of the chest and the stretch of the spine. Think inwardly of taking your head towards your feet (not to your knees, which will immediately hunch the back). It is much better to keep practising the lift of the chest, and the extension upwards of the spine to the crown of the head, until the spine has stretched enough to bring the chest flat down onto the thighs (main photo, this page). This may take months or years to achieve, but to keep the lift of the chest and the extension of the spine works much more effectively towards the final position than allowing the back to hunch. You can prac-

tise in the latter way for years without getting anywhere, as it constricts the spine and abdomen.

Once you are as far as you can go, take hold of the feet or whatever part of the legs you can, and relax there as long as you feel comfortable, breathing normally, as the posture is very restful and calming. In surrendering fully into the posture, it is very helpful to place blocks or a folded blanket on your legs for you to rest your head on, as shown in the upper photo at the right. This enables the busy mind to let go of its hold. As the head relaxes onto the support bring your awareness down to the belly and let the belly spread and relax onto the thighs. This allows the stretch of the spine to come much more from the base, over the sacrum. Check that you are not hunching the shoulders or pulling yourself forwards; the movement needs to come from the base of

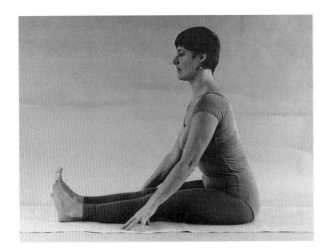

the spine to give a complete extension of the spine. Inhale to stretch the back up as shown in the photo above when you are ready to come up, then exhale and bring the spine right up.

POINTS TO WATCH AND WORK ON

1. The inner extension from the pubic bone to the chest is more important than pulling and hauling yourself forward with your arms and shoulders, which if done will tighten the shoulders and curve the spine; so if you feel any strain or hunching of the back, use a belt (as in the lower photo at right), as this helps the stretch of the spine. It will then extend forward without any effort. Continue to use the belt until the spine feels really stretched, and as you are able to move further forward, use a couple of blocks to rest the head on, rather than go into the hunched position.

2. If you have lower-back problems, sciatica, or unevenness in your hips, or if you are pregnant, do not go forward but stretch up with a belt around the feet, with the feet a hip-width apart.

3. If you feel that the lowest part of the spine tends to move backwards, rather than forwards over the legs, the legs are probably over-stretched at the knees, as explained for *uttana-*

sana; so let the knees bend a little and then the belly will be able to spread down onto the thighs more easily. This in turn will bring the base of the spine and the sacrum forwards.

EFFECTS

This posture lengthens and strengthens the spine, thereby increasing vitality by allowing the freer flow of energy up and down it. *Paschimottanasana* tones the abdominal organs and kidneys, improving the digestion. It rests and refreshes the mind and the emotions, bringing a deep inner peace.

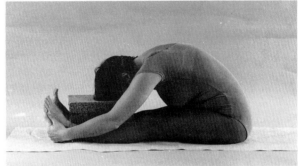

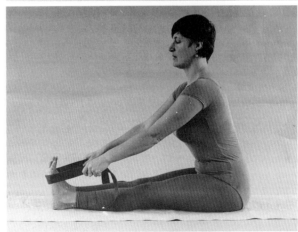

CHAPTER SEVEN

Backward-bending Postures

When the will to become Christlike grows strong in the heart, it causes an opening in the consciousness for the greater self to descend into the physical body. You think that your physical body is you, but it is only an infinitesimal part of you. If you would contact your true self, go into a place of quiet to commune with your Creator in your heart.

White Eagle, THE QUIET MIND

THESE ARE POSTURES which take the spine backwards, and thus wake up the whole system, giving a tremendous vitality and feeling for the joy of life. Yet they take you to that quiet place within, by opening the heart centre out, so that you can rise in consciousness. They give lightness of heart, overcoming any heaviness of the outer mind and outer body.

However, there is a great resistance in our spines to moving backwards, especially if we have hunched ourselves forward over desks or sinks or in cars for years. So the spine needs a little gentle yet firm persuasion to ease it into these postures, which is why it is very helpful to bend back over chairs or stools or beds, anything which supports the spine where it is weakest—that is, in

the lumbar region (the small of the back)—and move it where there is greatest resistance to movement—that is, in the upper back (dorsal spine). The mind also has a great resistance to back bends as they bring up many old fears, especially as we cannot see where we are going when we go backwards. Difficulties in backward-bending postures, including associated backaches, are generally due to lack of trust in ourselves, in others, in God. So the effect of working at the postures is to conquer fear, enabling us to trust the process of life and the God within, guiding us.

Always start with a few standing poses and then *uttanasana* or a few Dog poses (given at the beginning of chapter 10, the *Surya Namaskar*) before going on to backward-bending postures.

AWARENESS AND ATTENTION

Feel and concentrate on the opening of the heart centre, on the life and vitality this brings into the heart. Try to recognize any fear of going into these postures that you may have, especially those in which you go back and cannot see where you are going. Go through the fear when you are ready to, as that will bring tre-

mendous trust and confidence in God, in the universe, and its power to take care of you. After you come out of the posture, pause to become aware of the life and energy that now flows through your whole body, mind and spirit. These postures literally wake you up to life.

Setu Bandha Sarvangasana (Bridge Pose)

The Sanskrit name of this posture indicates that it is a variation on the Shoulder-stand, that opens out the chest in preparation for that pose; it lifts the mind in the heart above the mind in the head, so that the head-mind surrenders and lets go of its hold. The spine is very gently eased into a back bend in this posture.

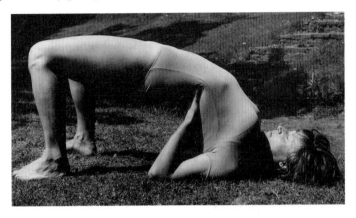

Lie flat on your back with knees bent, your feet parallel, hip-width apart and flat on the ground close to the buttocks (top photo, overleaf). Take a moment to relax your back onto the ground. Ease the shoulders down, ease your neck along the ground away from the shoulders. As you inhale take your awareness right down into your feet, spreading the toes and heels into the ground. As you exhale, stretch your knees away from you so that the thighs stretch out from the hips, and thus gently lift the hips and lower spine off the ground (middle photo, overleaf). Take several breaths to lift the spine to its maximum without strain, then link your hands together on the ground under your back, easing first one shoulder down and then the other (bottom left photo, overleaf). Taking your elbows in under your back, bend them to take your hands on to the sacrum (the flat bone in

the pelvis that joins to the lumbar spine). Stretch the sacrum and lower back away from you to lift the chest and relax the belly.

After you have been practising the posture for some while, and if the lower back is quite comfortable, take your hands higher up your back onto the ribs to lift the chest and heart higher, keeping the head and throat relaxed (main photo, this page). To come down, exhale, and stretching the base of the spine towards the feet let the back relax on the ground. If there is any strain in your back, bend the knees across your chest and put your arms around your legs to bring them towards you.

POINTS TO WATCH AND WORK ON

1. If there is any strain in your back or you are feeling at all tired or depleted, it is very helpful to find a low stool to lie over

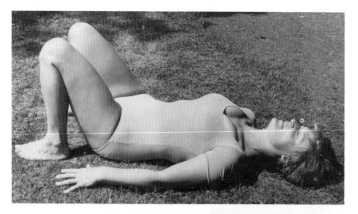

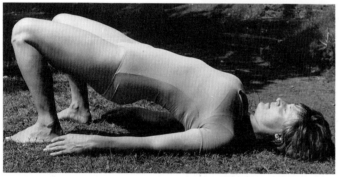

when doing this posture (photo below). It helps the spine to move where it needs to, stretches the neck, and the effect is very refreshing and revitalizing. Hold the position for four or five minutes when supported in this way.

2. Make sure the heels *feel* as though they are slightly turned out as there is always a tendency to bring the heels towards one another, which tightens and restricts the lower back and hips.

3. Keep the throat and head relaxed—come up from the feet and legs. If the throat and head tighten, do not go so far into the posture; keep the arms straight, as in the middle photo (left).

4. Allow the legs and *outer* hips to lift the spine, by stretching from the outer hips to the knees and down into the heels. This allows the belly to relax back onto the sacrum so that the spine is not then constricted. The ability to move into and maintain the posture comes from the extension in the thighs and heels so that the spine is not forcefully pushing itself into an arch but just naturally curves from the movement in the legs and hips.

EFFECTS
This posture opens the heart and chest, and helps the breathing especially for those with asthma or bronchial troubles. It lightens the heart and the spirits. It creates a flexible, strong spine which strengthens the nervous system.

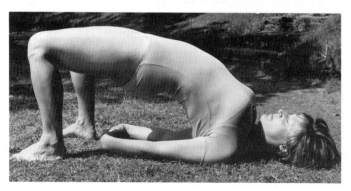

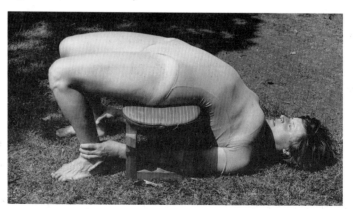

Urdhva Dhanurasana (Face-up Bow Pose or Back Arch)

Although this posture is the first of the more challenging backward bends, I have found that it is good to start working on it reasonably soon in your practice, perhaps after a year of work on the standing postures and forward bends, since it works much more on the whole spine than those postures known as the 'baby back-bends' such as the Cobra and Face-down Bow pose. Although the Cobra, for example, appears much easier to lift into, it is usually practised incorrectly at first, putting strain on the lower back while not moving the upper back: it is a much more advanced back bend than this one.

Do not be concerned if you do not seem to get very far; the attempt itself will begin to free the spine, the shoulders and the hips, bringing life and vitality to the whole body, mind and spirit. It is helpful to follow the instructions for the Bridge pose and practise it a couple of times to loosen up for this posture.

If your blood pressure is high or you feel any strain do not proceed with this pose without consulting a teacher.

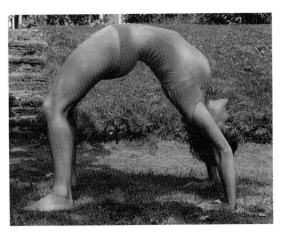

I : THE POSTURE OVER A CHAIR

This is a very good way to ease the spine into a back bend, as it moves and bends the dorsal spine, whilst relaxing and easing the lumbar spine. This is an area in which many people feel strain when doing back bends because they collapse into the lower back and resist movement in the upper back. The resistance of movement in the upper back comes from an armouring we place around our hearts for protection. We all do this to different extents: any hurt to the heart that we may have suffered in our lives makes us close up a little and protect ourselves from further hurts, and so we tend to 'close down' upon life's experiences and eventually shut ourselves away from the lessons we need to learn.

Back bends break through these defences and allow us to trust the process of life. The experiences it brings, even though hurtful, teach us the lessons we have come to learn. As White Eagle says, we are never given more than we can cope with and we are always helped and supported through trials, whether we know it or not; we just need to open ourselves to the awareness that we are looked after. Backward-bending postures help this, and the overcoming of these fears in back bends allows us to be open to give and receive love without fear of rejection.

Place a chair about two feet away from a wall, sideways on; sit sideways on the chair so that your toes are stretched up the wall, heels on the ground. The chair must have parallel sides; if it is a

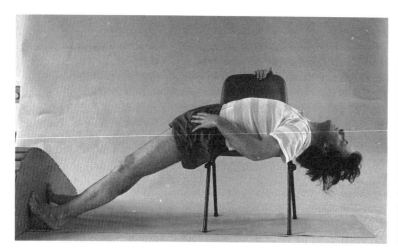
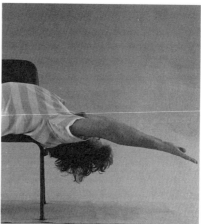
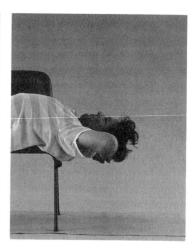

metal tube chair with canvas covering you can get into the back of it. Sit with the sacrum (the flat bone at the back of the pelvis joining on to the lumbar spine) just off the edge of the chair, so that the lumbar spine can stretch out from the sacrum. Keeping hold of the sides of the chair, go backwards over it so that the crown of the head is towards the ground behind you. Then press your feet against the wall so that you push the chair away from it and your legs straighten (above left).

If you are comfortable you can then take your arms over your head, stretching them away and towards the ground (central picture) or linking at the elbows; if there is any strain on your neck, link your hands behind your head to support it (right-hand picture). There should be *no* discomfort in your lower back: if there is, you are not in quite the right position—try moving the sacrum further down over the side of the chair to stretch the lumbar spine a little more, or roll a blanket lengthwise under the lumbar spine to support it. Relax there for a few moments. Then if you feel quite confident there move over the chair a little more until your hands come onto the ground, fingers pointing to the heels; then, taking your hands and feet firmly onto the ground,

lift yourself off the chair on an exhalation, moving your chest forward to come in line with your hands. Relax back onto the chair on an exhalation.

It is important to come up in the right way. Bend your knees to take your feet flat on the ground first. Take firm hold of the sides of the chair, lift your head and chest together to come up and then go forward between your legs while still sitting on the chair. Stay there bending forward for a few moments.

POINTS TO WATCH AND WORK ON

1. If you feel at all dizzy or there is any pulsing or pressure in your head, then come up and go forwards, staying in that position for several minutes until the pressure has gone. When the posture has this effect, however, it often means that you have held your breath from fear, so try again, remembering to breathe easily and to exhale as you go back.

2. Always keep the feet firmly on the ground, with the heels out so that the feet are parallel. This stabilizes and steadies you.

II: THE POSTURE FROM THE FLOOR

Lie on your back, preparing yourself as for the Bridge pose. On an exhalation, stretch the knees away, lift the hips, lower back and chest up (as in the photo on the left-hand side of p. 114). Pause as you inhale, relaxing the throat, head and belly; as you exhale, take the hands back and under the shoulders, fingers pointing towards the heels. Inhaling, lift your chest a little more, exhale and stretch your hands and feet into the ground to come up onto the crown of your head. Pause as you inhale, bringing the knees in and the elbows towards each other, lifting your chest even more as you exhale. Stretch the arms and legs to lift your head off the ground, straightening your arms and lifting your chest to come in line with your hands (as in the photo, below right). Hold the pose for as long as you can go on lifting and stretching up into it. To come down, lift your head to look up to the ceiling, bend your knees and elbows and gently stretch your back flat on to the ground. As you exhale, bring your knees across your chest.

POINTS TO WATCH AND WORK ON

1. If you feel strain in your lower back once in the pose, lift your heels off the ground and turn your heels out more and lift your chest more; then bring the heels down, turning them out even more as you do so. This will relieve the strain as it has the effect of spreading the sacrum out and opening out the lumbar region.

2. This posture seems to require great effort and exertion to start with, but if you can relax and extend into it and soften the whole body, particularly the head and belly, both beforehand and once you are there, it will not feel nearly such hard work, for the reason that you will not be working so much from the ego.

3. If you feel dizzy or have a headache, you have probably held your breath and not 'let go' into the posture. Take the posture a little more gently, making sure you exhale as you move. Also keep your head lifted in the pose without straining the throat; this in turn helps the lumbar spine to stretch.

EFFECTS

This posture brings great flexibility and strengthens the spine, tones up the heart and abdominal organs, and quietens the head-mind. It brings energy, awareness and vitality to the whole body, and lightness of heart, coupled with a deeper, inner, quietness. If it does not increase the energy level or quieten the head-mind it means that you are pushing and forcing the body from the level of the ego, holding your breath and straining. This is often a stage we need to be aware of and work through; or else we may be content to go over a chair for a while longer, coming back to it when we are ready.

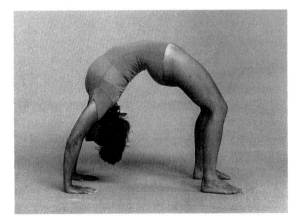

Ustrasana (Camel Pose)

This posture is said to bring enlightenment, because of the tremendous openness and lift it gives to the heart; it awakens the perceptions.

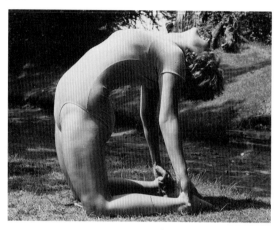

I : USING A WALL

Kneel down with your back to the wall so that your toes just touch it. Spread your heels a little apart, but not enough to make you sit between them; have the knees hip-width apart (photo opposite, left). If the buttocks do not feel relaxed in this position, sit on one or two blocks or books. Rest your head back against the wall and keep it relaxed there throughout the pose. Take your hands on to the soles of your feet, rolling your shoulders back towards the wall. Inhale, spread your chest out at the front and back; as you exhale, slide your head and chest up the wall and bring your thighs and hips forward in line with your knees. Then lift your chest away from the wall and up towards the ceiling, rolling the shoulders towards the wall even more (next photo). Do not push the lower back in or the belly forward: keep them spreading and

relaxed. Hold the pose as long as you can go on lifting the chest.

To come down, keep the lift of the chest, drop the thighs back and down on to the heels, and rest back into the wall.

Repeat this two or three times, then stretch forward and down on to the thighs, relaxing there (photo opposite, bottom right). When the chest lifts well and there is no strain on the lower back, try method II, the more traditional approach. Method I protects the lower back and neck from strain.

II : WITHOUT THE SUPPORT OF THE WALL

Kneel with the feet straight behind, the knees hip-width apart and the back up straight. Take your thumbs onto the sacrum and stretch it down towards the knees so that the lower back stretches out. As you inhale, lift the chest up; as you exhale, arch the spine

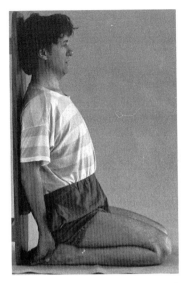
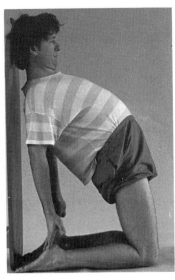
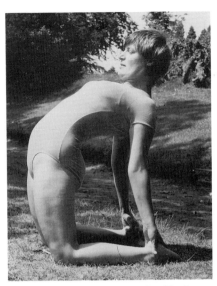

backwards as though you are taking the upper back, the dorsal spine, up and over a bar; keep the head lifted and the hips forward in line with the knees. When you feel that you are far enough back, take your hands on to your heels, roll the shoulders back and lift your chest up further. Do not constrict the neck by letting the head drop right back. Breathe easily in this position. Practise the pose for some while, keeping the head lifted a little until it can easily stretch out and back—the full position is illustrated on the first page. To come up, lift your head, chest and arms together as you exhale, sit back on your heels and then go forward over your legs, taking your head onto the ground (photo below right).

POINTS TO WATCH AND WORK ON

1. If the pose strains your lower back or neck do not take your head back but continue to have the wall behind you to support your head. Relaxing the belly, not pushing it forward, will relieve the lower back.

2. If you feel dizzy, or start to get a headache, again support your head against the wall and watch that you do not hold your breath.

EFFECTS

This posture relieves sluggishness, tones up the whole system, corrects a curved spine and hunched shoulders, and opens the heart centre, bringing joy and vitality.

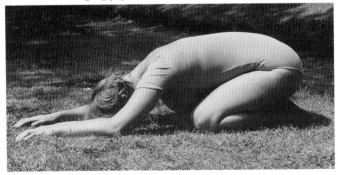

CHAPTER EIGHT

Inverted Postures

If you want to get a clear picture of any condition in life, don't try to see things with your nose on them! See them from the highest point, from the plane of spirit, and you will be surprised at how different your problems look.

White Eagle, THE QUIET MIND

POSTURES WHICH turn the whole body upside down have a great effect at all levels—rejuvenating the whole body, revitalizing all the internal organs, resting and refreshing the brain. At a mental level we are literally turning our world upside down—looking at all that worries and troubles us in a new perspective, thus enabling us to be a little less wrapped up in them.

The inverted postures help us to stand back a little, look from the highest point and detach ourselves from everyday cares. Inwardly they lift us up out of the heaviness of the earth, nearer to God, taking the feet—the understanding—nearer to heaven.

Always practise a few Face-down Dog poses (given at the beginning of chapter 10, the *Surya Namaskar*) or a few standing poses, and then *uttanasana*, the Standing Forward Bend, before starting on inverted poses.

CAUTION. Do not do these postures on your own if you have high or low blood pressure or any heart condition; if you have had an eye operation or detached retina or neck problems; or if they make you dizzy or the blood rushes to your head. In all these cases, consult an experienced teacher. Do not practise inverted postures during menstruation. Do not start to practise these poses if you are pregnant—or, if you are very used to doing them, let someone help you up and down in the later stages of pregnancy so that it's a gentle landing!

AWARENESS AND ATTENTION

Be aware of the tremendous increase in the flow of energy all around the system as a result of the body being upside down, the awareness that the body does not have to be dragged down by gravity but can lift itself up off the earth as though it could fly. Also be aware of the great sense of rest and relaxation given to all the organs of the body as a result of being upside down.

Salamba Sirsasana (Head-stand)

The Head-stand is known as the king of *asanas*. In yogic tradition, the brain is said to be the king of the body; and through the practice of standing on the head, the brain cells stay healthy and so control the rest of the body. This posture also stimulates the masculine principle giving courage, determination and strength—for this reason the Shoulder-stand should always be practised afterwards, as this stimulates the feminine principle, bringing balance of the inner energies.

You should have practised the standing postures and the Shoulder-stand (*salamba sarvanganasana*) for at least one year before attempting this important pose. Do not be in a hurry to go right up into the pose—spend some weeks or months on the preparation. If you try to achieve the full pose too quickly you might fling yourself up into it out of control instead of going up easily and gently in a balanced way. Make

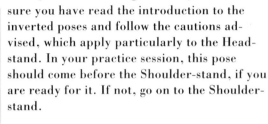

sure you have read the introduction to the inverted poses and follow the cautions advised, which apply particularly to the Head-stand. In your practice session, this pose should come before the Shoulder-stand, if you are ready for it. If not, go on to the Shoulder-stand.

I : PREPARATION

Fold a blanket so that it is wide enough to take the lower arms right to the elbow as shown in the picture. Kneel down and take your elbows onto the blanket, shoulder-width apart (no wider), linking the hands. The wrists should be firmly stretching down into the ground, the fingers firmly but not tightly clasped, the palms apart (overleaf, bottom left-hand photo). Do not think of going up into the posture yet—the preparation is to loosen the shoulders and stretch the neck out.

Keeping the shoulders spread and lifted, exhale, and stretch your back up as though for Face-down Dog pose (p. 146), keeping your head free of the ground; stretch the shoulders up and let the neck stretch down out of the shoulders (photo overleaf, top right).

If your head is off the ground, walk your feet in towards your elbows, keeping the base of the spine stretched up towards the ceiling; let the top of your head come lightly down onto the ground at the mid-point of the equal-sided triangle made by your lower arms (photo overleaf, lower right). Go on stretching your spine up and the legs back as though they are doing the Dog pose, until you reach the limit of your extension.

To come down, bend the knees and rest back onto the thighs. Keep the head down for a couple of minutes before sitting up.

IMPORTANT. If you feel heavy in your head, have difficulty in lifting your shoulders, or your neck feels at all constricted when bringing your head down, then just practise as far as the position of the upper right-hand photo until the shoulders feel more free and the neck stretched. This may take weeks or months, so do not be in a hurry.

2: TO GO UP INTO *SIRSASANA*

If you would like to have a wall, or a friend, behind, do so to begin with; but after some practice start to come away so that you do not become too dependent upon the prop. (If you are elderly and want to continue with the wall behind you, please do so.)

Go through the preparation. Keep the lift of the shoulders and the lift of the base of the spine and the back stretched up (right-hand column, lower photo). Go on lifting the base of the spine up until the knees bend and the feet come off the ground; exhale and then just steady yourself in this position (opposite, left-hand photo). Keep the chest moving forwards over the elbows, so that you do not roll over. (It does not matter if you do feel yourself going over—just release your fingers and roll and then start again. It is also good to learn to fall over as it takes away any fear.) Then on an exhalation stretch your legs up straight (main photo, p. 121, repeated right). Go on extending and stretching yourself up, extending the elbows down, extending the feet heavenwards, opening the soles of the feet to the light. Feel the energy coming down through them.

Only hold the pose as long as you can stay there without feeling

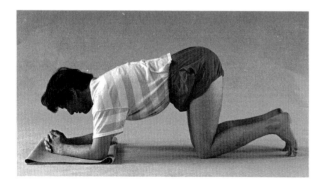

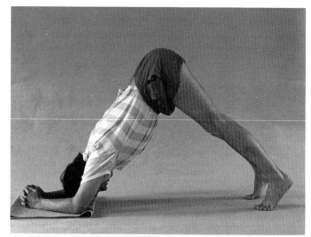

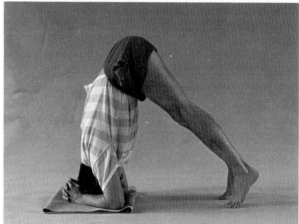

any heaviness on your head. Come down as you went up, on an exhalation, gently and under control. Keep your head down for a couple of minutes.

POINTS TO WATCH AND WORK ON

1. If you feel abnormal discomfort in your neck or head, or

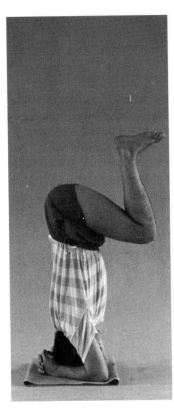
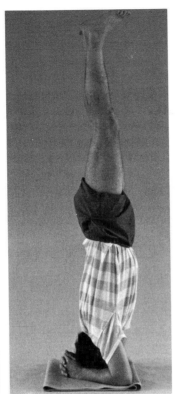

This posture brings steadiness of mind, and rejuvenates and adjusts the pineal and pituitary glands, and therefore all the glands of the endocrine system. It replaces lost energy, and is a great help for insomnia and nervous exhaustion and loss of memory as it increases the flow of blood to the brain so clearing the thoughts. It brings warmth and strength to the body, giving greater endurance. The combination of the Head-stand and the Shoulder-stand improves the haemoglobin content of the blood. They relieve colds, coughs, palpitations and constipation.

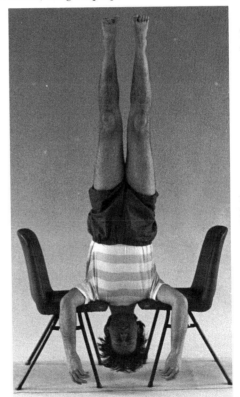

any dizziness or pressure, consult a teacher before continuing.

2. Watch that the back does not curve too much in the lumbar spine. To avoid this, lift the sacrum, spread the belly and waist back, the chest forwards. If you still feel curved or uncomfortable, try practising the posture on an outward-facing corner so that the spine can stretch up against the corner.

3. Another way to achieve most of the effects of the Head-stand is to rest the shoulders on two chairs with a gap in between for your head. This is particularly helpful if your neck needs a stretch or you feel heavy on your head (illustrated right).

Adho Mukha Vrksasana (Full Arm-balance)

Anyone who performed hand-stands as a child will remember the great delight, energy and confidence they gave. So why did we stop doing them? They will continue to give that same delight at whatever age we do them. It is good to practise this pose after the Face-down Dog pose and before or after the Head-stand. When practised first thing in the morning, the Full Arm-balance helps you instantly to become wide awake, ready to meet the day and whatever it brings to you. Many people find this pose comes more easily than the Head-stand, especially if there is a tendency to put too much pressure on the head, but generally start practising this pose when you feel happy in the Head-stand.

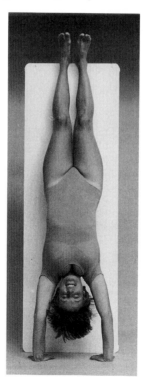

Have a wall behind you when first practising this pose. First stretch back into Dog pose with your finger-tips just two or three inches from the wall. Then walk in a little towards the wall, lifting up the base of the spine. Exhaling, swing one leg up and towards the wall, leting the other leg follow so that both legs now stretch up the wall, the head and neck extending down to the ground (see photo opposite). Remember to keep the arms firm and straight as you stretch yourself up against the wall, lifting the base of the spine and sacrum up the wall, easing the heels one by one up the wall, opening the soles of the feet out, opening the chest forwards and lifting out of the shoulders. Come down as soon as you lose that lift and extension upwards. Keep the head down in *uttana-sana* (Standing Forward Bend) for a while. Then repeat the pose with the opposite leg going up first. When this is mastered, bounce up with both legs.

POINTS TO WATCH AND WORK ON

1. If it is difficult to swing up into the pose at first, try and find a narrow corridor and walk up one wall until you can swing over to the opposite wall.

2. If you feel dizzy or heavy in the head, do not continue. Consult a teacher.

3. If your arms give way under you, practise the Dog pose for a while longer before attempting this pose again. The feeling of the arms wanting to give way actually stems from tightness in the shoulders, not lack of strength in the arms, so try opening the shoulders, out away from the spine.

EFFECTS

This pose brings instant energy, vitality, life and awareness. It strengthens the shoulders, arms and wrists and opens out the chest. It lightens the whole body and the spirits.

Salamba Sarvangasana (Shoulder-stand)

The Sanskrit *salamba* means 'supported'. *Sarv* means 'all', 'whole', 'entire', and *anga* means 'body' or 'limb'; therefore *sarvanga* means the entire body. Every part of the body at all levels benefits from this posture, which is one of the three main classical poses of yoga, together with *sirsasana* and *paschimottanasana*.

Salamba sarvanganasana is known as the mother of the *asanas* because it nurtures and cares for the whole system. While in this pose I am reminded of a bulb, nestled deep in the earth with the shoots sprouting up towards heaven. It emphasizes the feminine principle, that is, it stimulates the feminine energy within the body to encourage a sense of *being*, rather than forever *doing*—something that is very much needed in the western world! And so it brings peace, stability and security—like the role of the mother in the home. In this way it complements *sirsasana*—the Head-stand: the two work together to balance the energies in the body.

It is best to practise a few Dog poses, standing postures or forward bends each time before going into this pose.

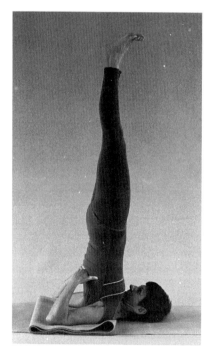

Lie flat on your back, allowing a moment or two for the neck to extend out of your shoulders, relaxing in the throat (photo opposite, top left). Ease the shoulders down and bring the arms to the sides. Gently inhale, and as you exhale bend your knees across your chest (next photo), ease your hands into the ground to lift the hips and lower back off the ground, then support your back with your hands (opposite, far right, top).

Take your feet onto the ground behind you in *halasana*, the plough pose (far right, middle

photo), which is the next posture given in this book (p.130). If this is at all difficult or any strain on your lower back, have a chair ready behind you to take your feet onto (far right, bottom) as you will then get much more stretch up in your spine, rather than the spine being curved.

Once your feet are on the ground or chair, behind your head, stretch your arms away from your head, linking your hands, easing one shoulder and then the other down away from

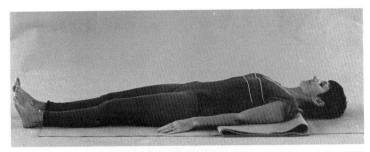

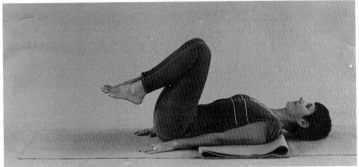

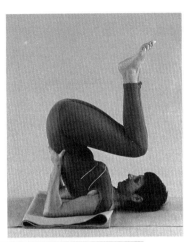

to it. When you are ready to come down, go into *halasana* (Plough pose, as in the two photos below) again, for a few moments. If you feel comfortable in the Plough pose go into the more relaxed version, relaxing the feet and the arms over the head (illustrated overleaf, lower left). Then, supporting your back, exhale, bend your knees and roll down, taking your hands onto the ground when you are almost down, for a light landing.

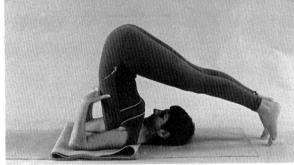

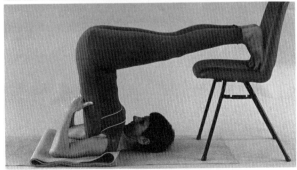

your ears (as in the upper left-hand photo on page 128). Then bend your elbows to support your back with your hands, as high up the ribs towards the shoulders as you can. Inhale, bend your knees; as you exhale, stretch your legs up towards the ceiling (main picture, opposite); feel as though your feet are doing the Mountain pose on the ceiling, so that they are neither pointed nor flat, but in-between. Open the soles out to receive the light. Go on stretching up towards the heavens, rolling your fingers over your ribs to lift your chest, aiming to have the whole body stretching up straight from the shoulders to the feet. Keep your throat and head relaxed, eyes looking towards your navel—literally contemplating your navel.

It is helpful to aim to hold this posture for at least four minutes, as that is the time it takes for the blood to recirculate completely; but do not strain to do so at first. Gradually build up

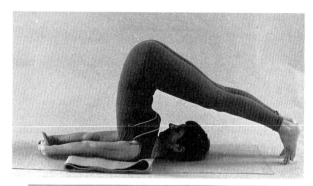

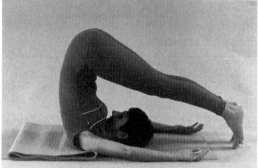

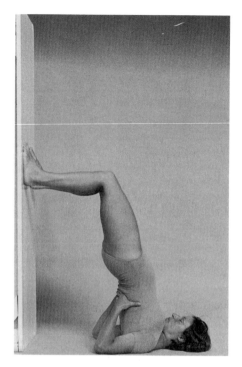

Rest there for a few moments.

Shoulder-stand is a very good prelude to *savasana*, relaxation, as it prepares and quietens the whole system, so make the most of that and go into your relaxation now.

POINTS TO WATCH AND WORK ON

1. If your neck feels seriously constricted or you feel any pressure in your head or buzzing in your ears in this pose, do not continue until you have consulted a teacher. If there is any more general strain on your neck or you feel heavy and uncomfortable, then try using the wall. Lie with your legs up the wall, your buttocks touching the wall. Inhale, bend your knees and push your feet firmly into the wall, heels turned out; exhale, lift your

back off the ground, supporting your back with your hands. Walk your feet up the wall so that your knees make a right angle. Keeping the lift of your chest, stretch your feet into the wall, to lift the hips in line with the shoulders (photo above). This has just as much benefit as coming right up, and it actually works the legs well, so keep your feet on the wall, just raising one leg at a time on an exhalation when you feel ready (opposite, top left). Exhale to bring the back onto the ground again and relax there for a few moments.

2. Another way to relieve the neck is to put a folded blanket or blocks underneath the shoulders. Leave the head free and make sure the elbows are on the block or blanket as well.

3. USING A CHAIR. If you feel that your chest collapses down and

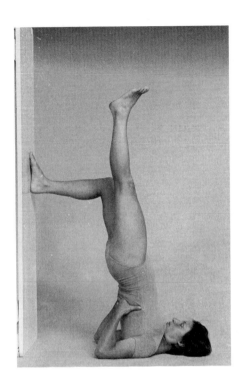

This posture calms the whole system by adjusting the functioning of the endocrine glands. It works particularly on the thyroid and parathyroid to regulate the metabolic rate. In this way, it also replaces lost energy. It clears the body of toxins so it is good to do when the body is at all infected (supported by a chair, or wall and blocks, so that the posture can be held comfortably if you feel weak). It has a beneficial, restorative effect on all the internal organs; it clears and calms the head, and prevents and cures headaches (unless caused by high blood pressure). It is particularly helpful after illness in restoring the whole system. It has a nurturing, mothering effect at all levels—emotionally, physically and spiritually.

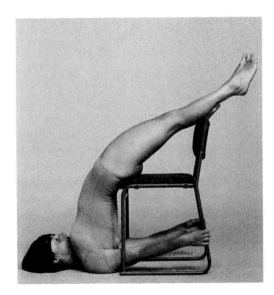

it is difficult to get a feeling of stretching upwards, then doing this posture with a chair is helpful.

To get into this pose, put a blanket over the chair and then start with your legs on the chair and your back on the ground. Take hold of the chair and, exhaling, go over into the Plough. Pull the chair in until it is touching your back. Bend your knees up and roll the sacrum over the seat of the chair to take your feet onto the back of the chair. If and when you are ready stretch your legs out over the back of the chair (right-hand photo).

Come down as you went up, exhaling. This is a very restful and refreshing way of doing the Shoulder-stand and is of great help in eventually achieving the full pose.

Halasana (Plough Pose)

This posture is named the plough because it resembles a plough that tills the earth, stimulating and reviving the soil, and this is the effect it has on the body. It is a very restful, comforting position when the body is ready for it.

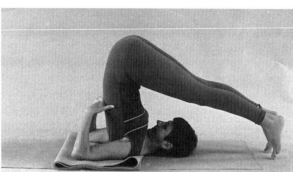

From the Shoulder-stand, keep the back supported with the hands; as you exhale, bend at the base of the spine and the buttock-bones. Take the legs down over the face so that the toes tuck under towards the head as they come down onto the ground (see photo on this page). Stretch the front of the thighs up and out of the hips, lifting the outer hips. If it feels too drastic a stretch on the lower back as you come down, then bend your knees over your face and then gradually stretch them out as far as they will comfortably go. Do not strain the back at all. If it is uncomfortable to take the feet right to the ground, have a block, or chair or stool ready behind you to take your feet onto (photo bottom right on p. 127). As you can see from these photos, you can actually lift the buttock-bones up higher, lengthening and straightening the spine much more if the feet are not taken so far down to the ground. Relax there for several minutes if it is comfortable to do so. To come down either roll the back ribs onto the ground, and bending the knees let the whole spine down onto the ground; or, supporting the back ribs, stretch back up into Shoulder-stand.

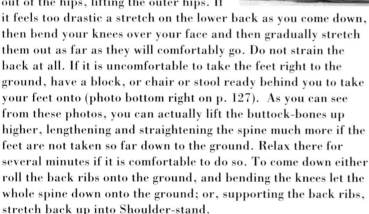

POINTS TO WATCH AND WORK ON

1. If the neck feels strained or the throat feels uncomfortable, putting the feet on a chair will help relieve this. Also place a blanket under the shoulders (as in the Shoulder-stand, Points to Watch, no. 2).

2. It is most important not to strain the lower back in this posture. If you have lower-back problems, or your hips are very uneven, or you have sciatica, do not practise this pose until the other poses have relieved the problem. Then go into it slowly, using a chair initially.

3. A more relaxed version of this pose, shown in the middle photo on p. 128, is to bring the tops of the feet onto the ground and take the arms towards the feet. Only go onto this version when you feel that you have mastered the one shown on p. 127, as this strengthens and lengthens the lower back until it can curve over into the other version without collapsing.

EFFECTS

The abdominal organs are rejuvenated by inverting and contracting them in this pose, which also has effects similar to those of *salamba sarvangasana*, the Shoulder-stand. It relieves backache, once the spine can extend into it: as stated in the introduction, postures which seem to trigger off or create pain or a problem are actually the postures which will cure the condition if practised in the correct way. It is helpful to those with high blood-pressure. If there is a rush of blood to the head in *sarvangasana* then go into *halasana* for a few minutes first, and *sarvangasana* will then feel much less of a strain on the head. *Halasana* also relieves wind (flatulence) and digestive problems, stiff shoulders and arms.

CHAPTER NINE

Seated Postures

He attains Peace, into whom desires flow as rivers into the ocean, which though brimming with water remains ever the same; not he whom desire carries away.

BHAGAVAD GITA, Chapter II

The seated postures release the energy held in the hip-joints and sacrum—that is, in the basal and sacral centres—in a gentle, safe way, because of the stretch upward of the spine; and they allow that energy to move up to the brow and then balance in the heart. This movement of energy up and down the spine has the effect of release and relaxation in the busy outer mind. So the thoughts can come and go without the whole system being disturbed and thrown by them. Those restless, changing thoughts are 'put in their place' rather than being allowed to 'run riot' through our consciousness.

All the *asanas* in yoga work towards sitting: that is, being able to sit comfortably for meditation without the body protesting. However, it is as well to remember that the protestations, aches and pains in the body are not separate from the meditation but the beginning of it. Patanjali, the father of yoga, when giving instructions for meditation says in his *sutras* on 'How to know God': 'Sit in any comfortable *asana*'. He was taking it for granted that this is perfectly possible and easy; yet a western body can take years to feel comfortable in the seated postures. Moving from one seated posture to another frees the hips, knees and ankles so that we can then sit more easily with the spine straight. This enables the energy to be balanced up and down the spine from the base to the head—the centre being the heart—and so quietens the mind ready for meditation. It is helpful to stretch the spine fully in the Dog pose, or standing poses, before doing these postures. *Parvatasana*, from the chapter on forward-bending postures, is also very helpful to include among the seated poses.

AWARENESS AND ATTENTION

While sitting in these postures, be aware of the peace and quietness they bring, especially to the brain, the mind in the head. Because they increase the flow of energy from the hips, the base of the spine and the sacrum, the blood—and therefore energy—is drawn down more into the body from the head so that we become aware that the divine life-force resides in every cell of the body.

Virasana (Hero Pose)

The pose is called 'hero' because it stimulates the inner fire in a controlled and safe way, giving heroic qualities of steadfastness and courage. It is very important for emotional control as it both frees and brings control to the diaphragm. This may seem a contradiction, but if emotion is held in and suppressed it can sometimes break out uncontrollably. The freeing of the diaphragm releases held-in emotion, so this posture can occasionally bring tears and strong feelings. Once these are released and the need to hold them in is no longer felt, the posture can bring control of the emotions, without suppression.

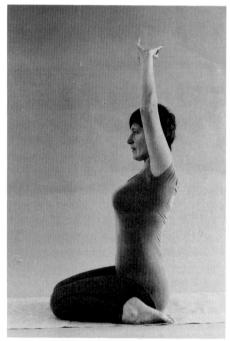

Sit on the knees and rest the buttocks back on the heels for a moment. Then separate the feet, turn the calves out with your thumbs (keeping the toes stretching straight back from you and spreading out) and sit down between the feet. If, as is usually the case at the beginning, it is not possible to come right down to the ground, then sit on a block, book or firm cushion so that you can

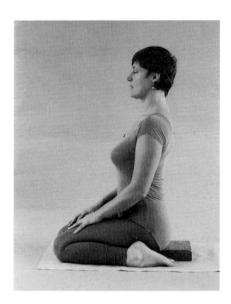

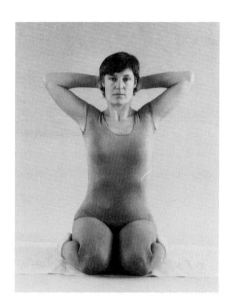

relax there. Do not cause any strain to the knees. Stretch the spine up through the centre (left-hand photo), with the hands just resting on the thighs and spreading the back and front of the body evenly, so that you are not pushing the lumbar spine in and the belly out. Then, link your hands and take them behind your head (right-hand photo); spread from the centre of the chest to the elbows, inhaling; as you exhale, turn the palms towards the ceiling and stretch your arms overhead (main photo, opposite page). Hold the position as long as you can stretch up into it; exhale to come down, keeping the lift of your chest.

Change the link of the hands so that the opposite index finger is on top: this will feel very odd at first but is important for balance. Then repeat the stretch of the arms.

EFFECTS

This posture quietens and calms the whole body, and the emotions, mind and nervous system; it frees the hip, knee and ankle-joints, and enables the breath to deepen right down to the diaphragm and abdomen, so unblocking the solar plexus. It relieves bronchial and asthmatic conditions and nervous tension, and is helpful during pregnancy. It takes one down to the centre of one's being, as it opens the heart centre.

Supta Virasana

This extension of *virasana*, lying back down behind, opens the diaphragm and chest even more and is very relaxing and refreshing but you should not rush into it, since the lumbar spine needs first to be well extended out of the sacrum so that there is no constriction. If you are new to this posture when you read this book, just do *virasana* for the first few weeks or months.

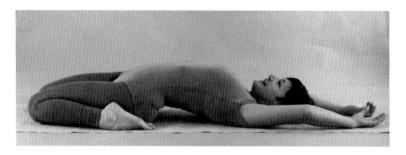

From *virasana*, take your hands onto the ground a few inches behind the toes, with fingers pointing towards the toes. Inhale, lift your heart up, opening the chest out, and roll your shoulders back (left-hand photo opposite). Exhale, and bend your elbows so that you go back down towards the ground behind you.

If there is any strain in your back or your knees come off the ground, come up and put some sort of support (blocks or one or two blankets folded lengthwise) under your back as in the photo top right overleaf, so that your back can comfortably spread onto the support.

If you can relax right down onto the floor, spread the upper back between the shoulder blades, and the back of the neck out on the floor, then relax there for several minutes, with the arms down by your side; for more of a stretch, place the arms on the floor over your head (main photo, this page).

To come up, lift your head and chest together as you inhale, then as you exhale lift up and over to bend forwards. Bring the feet in to sit on the heels; separate the knees, then go forwards between the knees (lower photo on the right, opposite). Rest there for a few moments, then ease the legs back into the Dog pose and then give them a forward stretch into *dandasana*.

POINTS TO WATCH AND WORK ON

1. If the knees tend to be painful in *virasana*, make sure you have stretched them well beforehand, with standing poses or Dog poses, and sit on a block or two. Sit high enough for any pain in the knees to be relieved; you will gradually stretch and relax them there, and so with practice will gradually be able to sit lower down. If you try to sit right down too soon you will tend to tighten the knees and thigh muscles and may damage your knees.

2. Similarly, in going back into *supta virasana*, if you are not able to relax down into it you will strain and tighten the back, but if you have enough support so that you can relax there, you will eventually be able to release the lumbar spine out of the sacrum to enable you to lay the upper back down onto the ground. There will always be a curve in the small of the back because of the angle of the pelvis to the ground, but it needs to be an open curve, not jammed into the sacrum.

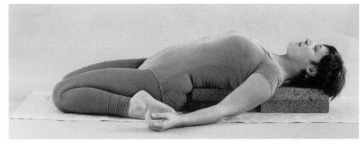

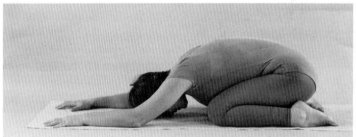

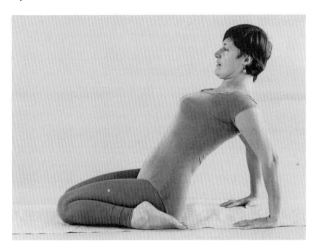

Baddha Konasana (Cobbler Pose)

Baddha konasana translates literally as the 'caught-angle' pose, but is known as the Cobbler pose since this is how Indian cobblers sit, with the shoe between their feet so that both hands are free. It is suitable for meditation (sitting against a wall) as it frees the hips and the base of the spine allowing the energy to travel freely up and down the spine, provided the spine is straight. This free movement of the energy helps to still the outer mind and brings the awareness to the mind in the heart.

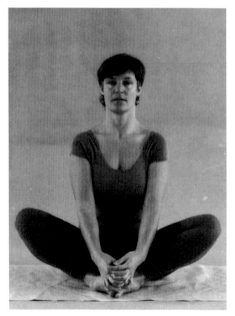

From *dandasana*, keeping the spine stretched up straight, bring the soles of the feet together, as close to the body as is comfortable. Take hold of the feet, as in the photo, or the ankles or shins, whichever feels best for you; just ensure that the spine remains straight and the shoulders do not hunch forward. Do not push the knees down; just allow the thighs to release out of the hip-joint and stretch away to the knees. Sit quietly extending the spine upwards, opening the chest out, bringing the side ribs forward and shoulders back, for three to five minutes, and then stretch the legs out.

With practice, this posture can be held longer, and is then a good posture for meditation.

POINTS TO WATCH AND WORK ON

1. If you have difficulties in stretching the spine up, sit flat against the wall; you may need a folded blanket or support in the back if the spine caves back into the wall: place the support just below the curve, then lift up and over it to spread the shoulders back to the wall (see photo below).

2. SUPTA BADDHA KONASANA. It is also helpful to practise the Cobbler pose lying down, particularly with the feet into the wall, as this releases strain in the groin. Begin as before, and spread the toes apart against the wall but have the soles of the feet together. Take the buttocks in close to the heels, then lie down, relaxing the sacrum, lumbar spine and belly back towards the ground (see photo below). Again, do not try to push the knees down as this causes strain in the back and abdominal organs, but do allow the thighs to release from the hips. After you have maintained the posture for a while you can feel if one hip releases more than the other: bring your awareness to the tighter side to let it go a little more. When you are ready to come out of the posture, take your hands to the outside of your knees to bring them together.

EFFECTS

This posture frees the sacrum and pelvic joints and rejuvenates the abdominal organs; it relieves sciatica, urinary and genital disorders, and keeps the kidneys healthy. If practised regularly during pregnancy, it is very helpful to the labour. Together with the Hero pose, it safely and gently helps to integrate what is held subconsciously in the lower chakras with the conscious mind, the head-mind, making the point of balance the heart and thus helping to centre the awareness there.

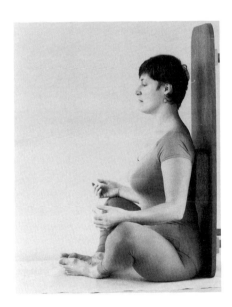

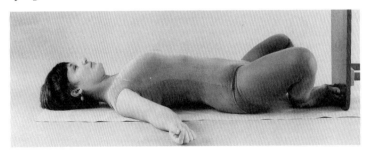

Siddhasana

A *Siddha* is a holy, mystical being who possesses *siddhis*: supernormal powers, such as the ability to levitate and to be in two places at once, and the perception to see the truth in all beings.

    Regular, daily practice of this posture develops the perceptions in this way, without allowing the misuse or the concentration in these powers for their own sake, but to further the evolution of mankind.

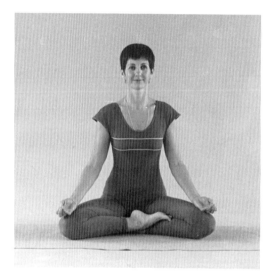

Sit in *upavistha konasana*. If the pelvis tilts back and the lower back feels curved, sit on a block, book, or firm cushion. Take the index fingers under the left knee (either side) to open the joint out as you bend it. Bend the left knee out to the side to bring the left heel into the groin, turning the sole of the foot upwards. Then take the fingers under the right knee to bend the knee, thus setting the heel of the right foot in line with the left, on the ground just in front of the left foot.

    Take your hands onto the ground behind you and stretch your spine up (photo, opposite page), relaxing the thighs out of the hips and the knees towards the ground. Stay in this stage of the pose if your knees are high off the ground.

    If your knees are relaxing down to the ground, bring the right foot up onto the left calf, still keeping the heels in line (main photo, above); then bring the wrists to rest on the knees, and stay there for at least three minutes (it is an ideal posture for meditation). Return to *upavistha konasana* and then repeat, this time bringing the right leg in first.

POINTS TO WATCH AND WORK ON

1. Do not be tempted to force and push the knees down as they will only bounce back and tighten, and you could damage the knee-joint. When the muscles are forced to extend they will then contract back to a tighter position than they were in before, whereas if you gently ease the thigh-bone out of the hip-joint and relax the knees, allowing just the weight of the wrist to gently ease them down, then they will gradually release.

2. The stretch up and straightening of the spine is much more important than getting the knees down to the ground. In fact the more you stretch the spine, the more the hips will release their tight hold on the thighs. If the spine feels curved, then sit flat back against the wall.

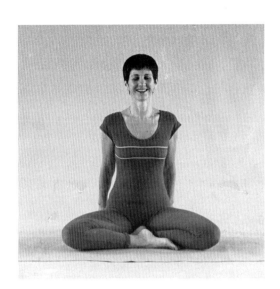

EFFECTS

Siddhasana has a quietening, calming effect on the mind and the emotions, allowing you to let go of the outer self and touch the Inner, Higher Self. It is inspiring and aspiring; regular practice enables one to keep in touch with the higher spheres and develop the intuition.

Preparation for *Padmasana* (Lotus Pose)

Padmasana is one of the classical and best-known postures of yoga. It is the pose most recommended for meditation because it provides a very firm, stable base for sitting and allows the spine to be absolutely straight and lengthened. This is, of course, so long as you do not force your body into it too soon, for then *padmasana* can have the reverse effect, that of over-stimulating the base centres in a dangerous and uncontrolled way, and of bringing about curvature of the spine, so trapping the energy that needs to flow freely up and down the spine in meditation.

It is likely to take many years (or many lifetimes) of practice of the standing postures and the two seated postures

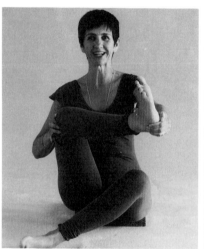 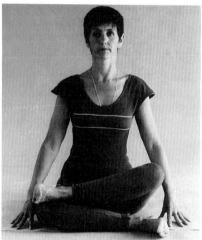

already given, as well as a good long while spent on the preparation, before achieving the full posture. However, if we let go of the idea of having to get into the full posture and be content to work on the preparation, gradually letting go into it rather than forcing into it, then the freedom it gives in the hips and sacrum creates the letting-go in our egos and structure of our lives. We need to be willing to let go in these areas to achieve this posture—an example of where the real inner effect of yoga comes in.

The sacral and base centres relate to our attitudes to our life-force or sexuality. The inner fire which is often equated with sexual energies is our creative life-force and stirs within our bodies, within the earth and the whole of nature in spring, creating life and beauty. These areas are also to do with our sense of security and trust in life, in God and the Inner Self. I often feel that the reason western bodies can have seemingly immovable rigidity in the hip-joint, sacrum and base of the spine, is the lack of understanding and fear of the real essence of these energies.

Our tendency is to put our security into houses, mortgages, investments, insurance, and so on, and cling onto other people rather than to trust the flow of the Universe. We see sexuality as an energy which either needs satisfying at a base level or suppressing as being immoral and unclean, rather than as a beautiful expression of a creative life-force, a path to at-one-ment with another person's Higher Self. As a result of our conditioning of fear, the sacrum and base vertebrae actually fuse together and become rigid in our early twenties.

The medical profession accepts that this happens, but because it is a conditioned response, it is actually possible to undo it through the postures of yoga and through meditation. It needs willingness, however, to let go of all that we 'hold onto for dear life'—the expression itself demonstrates the fear. Holding on, moreover, always manifests as pain— deep inner pain that needs to be experienced and worked through. You will know that this pain is good pain and to be experienced when you feel it, as you would have felt it when going forward in *parvatasana* (in the chapter on forward bends) which is a very good preparation for this pose. These postures cannot be undertaken lightly as they will create many internal changes, a loosening of the outer ego's hold and a deep inner searching. So spend a good long while on all the others, particularly *parvatasana*, *virasana* and *baddha konasana* and the standing postures, before going onto this preparation.

Starting in *dandasana*, bend the left knee and bring the shin-bone parallel to the line of your hips and to your mat or blanket under the right leg, keeping the heel extended, as this opens the hips; do not tuck the foot in, as in most 'lazy' ways of sitting cross-legged, because this puts strain on the ankles and knees and closes in the hips. The shin needs to be away from the hip; you will feel the opening in the hip when you are in the correct posture (the left-hand photo shows the right position of the left leg.)

Then take hold of the right foot with your left hand, stretching the heel into the hand (same photo), and place the heel and ankle-bone on top of the left knee, so that the right shin is over the left. The right knee is now immediately above the left heel so that you make a squarish shape. Stretch your spine up and back out of the hips, stretching the thighs forward away from the hips, leaning slightly back on your hands behind you. This position is shown in the right-hand photo, only with the legs the other way round.

It is helpful to keep moving the spine in this posture as this helps in letting go, so keeping the lift of the spine twist slowly first to the right and then to the left; and then go forward over the right knee, then to the centre, and next over the left knee. When going forward, pause with the inhalation, taking the breath into the hips; move forward out of the hips with the exhalation. Then change the legs around the other way, the right underneath and the left on top, and repeat the spinal movements.

It is helpful to change around two or three times, holding the positions longer and moving from side to side the third time. Then stretch your legs and go forward into *paschimottanasana*, the Sitting Forward Bend, to stretch your legs out.

POINTS TO WATCH AND WORK ON

1. If it feels that this posture is impossible, and your top knee is right up in the air and it throws you back, curving the spine, then leave the pose until you have practised the others for longer; it would also be helpful to sit on a block or two.

2. There should be no pain in the knees and ankles, just extension. If there is pain, stretch the ankles away more and bring the knees in towards each other.

Padmasana and *Ardha Padmasana* (Full Lotus and Half Lotus Poses)

After spending some considerable time on the preparation, and the other postures recommended for working towards *padmasana* (this may be weeks, months or years) you may feel ready to go into the Full Lotus or the Half Lotus. Do not rush to go into them—the preparation is as important, if not more important, than the full pose. It is the journey that matters, not the destination. As has already been stated, but cannot be over-emphasized, if you push your body into the Lotus before it is ready there can result much damage to the knees, leg muscles and ankle-joints, and you will also impede the flow of energy up and down the spine. Although it is recommended as the ideal posture for meditation in yogic texts, that is not taking into account the very stiff western hips. So for some time you need to be content with simply sitting cross-legged, in *baddha konasana*, or *virasana*. *Padmasana* will come when the whole body, inwardly and outwardly, is ready to release the blocks mentioned in the section on preparatory poses.

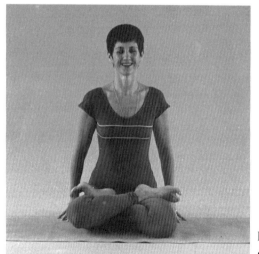

First, go into the preparatory pose (previous pages) and repeat two or three times on each side; then come back to the side with the left knee bent and the right leg on top. Keeping the heel stretching away over the left leg, gently bring the right leg up towards the hips, so that the right foot comes up to the root of the left hip, still keeping the heel well stretched away so that it is well up over the left thigh. This is the Half Lotus pose (photo opposite, left).

If the right knee can relax down near to the ground in this position, then you can bring the left foot out and onto the top of the right thigh, gently easing the foot up to the root of the thigh (photo opposite, right). Stretch your spine up, breathing normally, resting the hands on the thighs. This is the

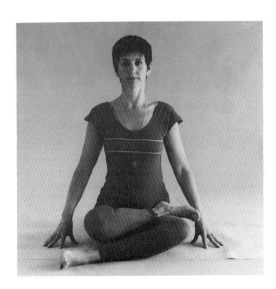

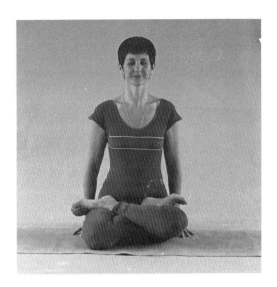

Full Lotus pose—*padmasana* (main photo, left-hand page).

This seems a more difficult way to get into the pose than is sometimes given, but it ensures that the hips are ready and that there is no damage to the knees. Stay as long as comfortable and then change the legs to the other way round. If you use this posture for meditation, it is not necessary to keep changing the legs in one meditation, but over a period of time check that there is balance by doing it one way and then the other.

POINTS TO WATCH AND WORK ON

1. If the knees are painful and the feet tend to fall into the groin it does indicate that the hips are not yet quite ready for the full pose; but try taking the hands to the outside of the knees and bring the knees in towards one another; this brings the feet more over the top of the thighs, and also gives more movement in the hips. If this does not take the pain from the knees, come out of the pose and practise the preparation for longer.

2. If you feel as though you cannot stretch your spine up straight, again you are pushing the legs into the pose too soon. A straight, extended spine is of utmost importance for energy balance, harmony and ease in the body—much more important than pushing yourself into this posture—so practise the postures in which the spine does feel extended and then come back to this one to see if you can keep the same extension. If you cannot, leave it for a while longer.

EFFECTS

The Lotus pose frees and tones the hip, ankle and knee-joints. It stimulates the circulation of the blood in the lumbar region of the spine, and this rejuvenates the spine and abdominal organs. It is recommended for meditation because freeing the base of the spine and sacrum in this way balances the energy along the spine, thus quietening the outer mind in the head and bringing the awareness into the heart, the centre of balance between the two points, the base and the crown.

CHAPTER TEN

Surya Namaskar and Dog Poses

We would be happy to see you all dancing a divine dance! We do not want to see you with solemn faces: we like to see you merry, we assure you that brothers on our side of life are not long faced. They have learnt to give joy to life, and in their giving they also become joy and happiness. In the brotherhood of ages past there was always to be found the spirit of happiness and fun; but remember, this brings wisdom and balance. It is so important to be balanced in your spiritual life. You may devote your life to spiritual service, but this doesn't mean a life of gloom. No—you radiate joy and light.

White Eagle, THE STILL VOICE

Surya Namaskar (Salutation to the Sun)

THIS BEAUTIFUL sequence of postures, designed to be practised at dawn, awakens the whole body, mind and spirit to greet the rising sun, to pay homage to the sun and to mother earth. It is like a divine dance lifting the spirits to God, to the sun, bringing joy and happiness.

There are twelve mantras to the sun, as follows:

1. Aum Hram Mitraya Namah (*mitro* = friend)
2. Aum Hreem Ravaya Namah (*ravi* = shining)
3. Aum Hroom Suraya Namah (*surya* = beautiful light)
4. Aum Hraim Bhanawe Namah (*bhanu* = brilliant)
5. Aum Hraum Khagaya Namah (*khaga* = who moves in the sky)
6. Aum Hrah Pushne Namah (*pushan* = giver of strength)
7. Aum Hram Hiranyagarbhaya Namah (*hiranyagarbha* = golden-centred)

8. Aum Hreem Mareechaye Namah (*mareechi* = lord of dawn)
9. Aum Hroom Adityaya Namah (*aditya* = son of aditi)
10. Aum Hraim Savitre Namah (*savitr* = beneficent)
11. Aum Hraum Arkaya Namah (*arka* = energy)
12. Aum Hrah Bhaskaraya Namah (*bhoskara* = leading to enlightenment)

I have not translated the first two and last words of the mantra. They create what is known as a *beeja* mantra: that is, evocative sounds which create a vibration in the body but may not have any actual meaning. The effect of chanting them is to concentrate and channel the mental energy so releasing tension in the mind. If you are unused to chanting mantras, but want to use them whilst practising *surya namaskar*, try choosing one that appeals to you, either chanting it internally to yourself or out loud if it does not make your breathing too strained.

Experiment a little to see how the mantras sound and feel, and the effects of chanting them. Various ways of using them are possible, but I suggest making a choice of one at a time and using it throughout the whole *surya namaskar*. It is not, however, necessary to use them to obtain the effects of *surya namaskar* if you are not comfortable with them.

According to ancient Hindu tradition each should be chanted nine times, which would give 108 complete sequences of the postures if you used one mantra for each sequence—something which would seem rather difficult for us to achieve in our busy lives! But it's a good idea to do four, six or twelve repetitions. You do not need to change the mantra, and if they are unfamiliar to you stick with one for each practice session. When going through several repetitions the salutations can be practised very fast, which stimulates the whole system, ready for the day. But when using the mantras the sequence needs to be practised more slowly and rhythmically to bring into them the feeling of opening to the sun, particularly in the solar plexus area, and then bowing down to the earth.

As we saw in Part One, the postures of yoga are found in the absolute balance point between strength and suppleness, so developing both. The *surya namaskar* sequence emphasises this: practised too slowly it can become lazy, lethargic and possibly head-orientated, practised too fast it becomes stiff and straining. So gradually find your own rhythm, in tune with the rhythm of your breath.

It is better to loosen up a little beforehand with Dog pose, so instructions have been given for the Face-up and Face-down Dog poses first, as they are often practised on their own. If you are just beginning the practice of yoga, it is better to work on the standing postures for a while and then work on the two Dog poses before attempting the whole sequence, as it is more demanding than is usually recognized. It is better to wait until it can come without strain; if there is any strain, leave the full *surya namaskar* for a while and just go through the other postures until it comes more spontaneously, giving to you the joy of living.

INTRODUCTION TO THE WHOLE SEQUENCE

There are several different versions of the *surya namaskar*, and this may be a slightly different one from those you have come across before—there is rather more extension to it and it avoids collapsing on the ground in the middle. I like the greater extension and have found it the most enlivening version, so I usually teach the *surya namaskar* in this way.

Do take the whole sequence at your own pace, in line with your own breathing rhythm.

Do not hold your breath at all. If you need to take extra breaths from the ones I have given please do so, always moving on an exhalation.

AWARENESS AND ATTENTION

Be aware of the very precise, deep, definite movements in each part of this sequence, and of the awakening they bring deep into the whole system all the way through to the spirit rising up to greet the sun. Be aware of the sun, the light in the heart, gradually becoming one with the spiritual sun, within the physical sun, as you go through the sequence.

Preparation: *Adho Mukha Svanasana* (Face-down Dog Pose)

Adho means 'down'; *mukha* means 'face', and *svana*, 'dog': so the Sanskrit means just the same as the English.

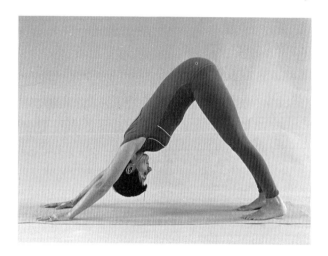

Sit on your knees, which should be slightly apart, resting back on the heels; on an exhalation lay the belly and chest on the thighs and head on the ground. Relax there for a moment, letting the forehead spread on the ground. Spread the ribs and belly on the thighs and the buttock-bones onto the heels (top right-hand photo). Then, stretching your arms forward, spread your hands and fingers out on the ground, shoulder-width apart (not closer), and come forward onto all fours and tuck the toes under (lower right-hand photo). As you exhale, lightly lift your hips high, lifting the heels and turning the tail-bone (coccyx) upwards as though you really do have a tail. Then stretch the thighs back and away out of the hip-joints and the heels away and down towards the ground so that the legs feel strong and are stretching you up

and back. Stretch the hands down and out on the ground so that the shoulders and shoulder blades spread apart and the spine can then go on stretching up (photo above). Hold the position just as long as you can. Stretch up into it breathing normally (come down before you feel heavy, as though you are just holding on), then exhale and relax down on the knees. Rest there for a few breaths and then repeat the pose two or three times.

It is helpful on the second or third time to ease up into the hips separately, by stretching the fingers of one hand and the toes of the foot of that same side down into the ground: this frees the back, hips and shoulders a little more. Then both hands and feet are able to stretch more firmly down into the ground, so that the spine stretches up more and the back can broaden and open out.

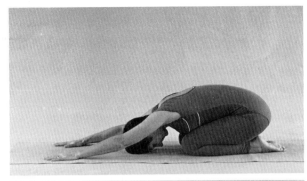

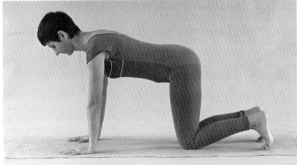

no. 1, so that the heels are a little more lifted from the ground. Then you will be able to work the legs more.

EFFECTS

This posture imitates the dog; like much of the animal kingdom, dogs fully and completely release and extend their whole body to bring life and awareness to every part. Just watching dogs or cats fully stretch themselves in the totally relaxed way they do gives the feeling of suppleness, aliveness and alertness. So practice of the Dog pose can have the same effect on us humans, who have lost so much of the natural movement that animals have. It relieves exhaustion, arthritis of the shoulders and hips, stiffness across the shoulder blades; it strengthens the ankles and knees, relieves aches from walking and running, slows the heart, strengthens the abdominal muscles and lengthens the spine. It is a good alternative to *salamba sirsasana* (Head-stand) if you are unable to do that, giving many of the same benefits, as the head and trunk are inverted.

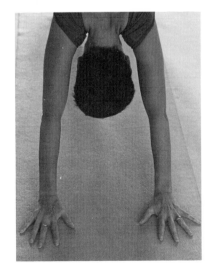

POINTS TO WATCH AND WORK ON

1. The distance of the hands from the feet is important and should be as in the photo to the right. The arms need to be stretched fully forward before you come up: if you keep that distance it gives a good stretch. If your hands and feet are too close together, the spine will be curved.

2. Do not let the heels come down heavily, as the ankle bones would then tend to collapse into the feet: stretch the shin bones up as well as back, the heels always stretching away, the toes forward. If the heels do collapse to the ground, have the feet and hands a little further away from each other than described in note

Urdhva Mukha Svanasana (Face-up Dog Pose)

It is helpful to practise Face-down Dog poses for a few weeks before going on to this pose, as the spine needs to be fully extended before arching.

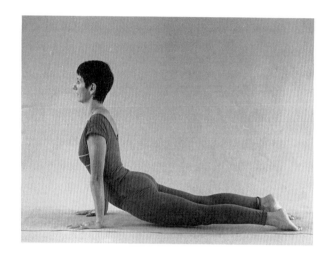

Follow the preceding instructions into the Face-down pose, and then from that exhale, lift your head, and bring your chest forward (the photo opposite, top, shows the beginning of this forward movement), rolling your shoulders back. Keep the legs stretching as though they want to stay back, so that the lower back stays stretched and the buttocks are relaxed (opposite, bottom). Lift your chest up by stretching firmly down on the hands, stretching the fingers, so that the shoulders can spread out and back, keeping the neck and head in line with the back (same photo). If you can comfortably do so, roll over the toes onto the top of the feet: this lifts the trunk forward and up more (main photo, this page). The thighs should be just off the ground, the shins lifting. Exhale, go back into the Face-down Dog pose when you are ready, and then relax down you began that pose, shown in the top picture on p. 147.

POINTS TO WATCH AND WORK ON

1. If the lower back feels compressed and uncomfortable, it is due to the belly pushing forward and straining. Take your awareness down into the belly and think of lifting it and spreading it out into the hips and the lumbar spine; stretch the legs away out of the hips to the heels, turning the heels out to the sides to open and free the sacrum.

2. If the neck is uncomfortable, do not take the head back, but spread the chest and shoulder blades out and the shoulders down, and let the back of the neck stretch out of the shoulders, the crown of the head pointing straight up, throat relaxed.

EFFECTS

As with the Face-down Dog pose, this pose gives the full extension that a dog achieves and the effects of release and life. Practising the two together releases the spine and the hip-joints and helps the blood to circulate freely; it loosens the shoulders and upper back, relieving backache, stiffness and tiredness, and giving the feeling of joy, vitality and aliveness.

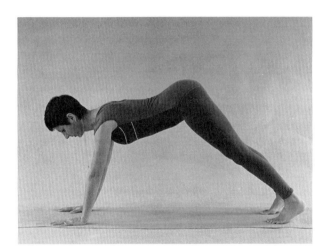

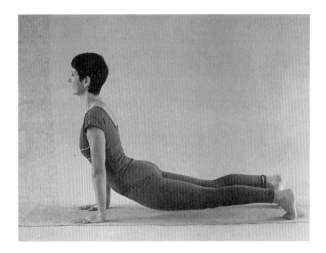

Surya Namaskar—whole sequence

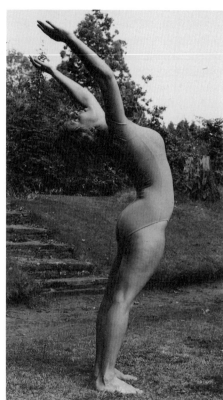

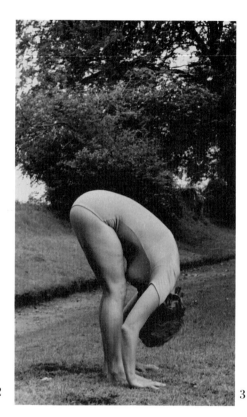

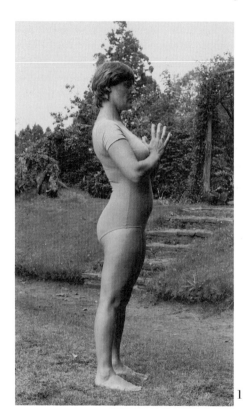

Stand in *tadasana* (Mountain pose), with the hands together in *namaste* (prayer position) over the heart (photo 1). Just spend a moment centering yourself in the heart, quietening the head.

Inhaling, stretch your arms up over your head, exhale, arch the spine backwards by stretching the heels into the ground, lifting the heart up to the sun, looking upwards (photo 2). Inhale to come upright; exhaling, bend forward from the hips into *uttanasana*, taking the hands to the ground beside the feet (photo 3). If you need to bend the knees, do so, keeping the buttock-bones lifted: it is much better to have the knees a little bent than locked back, so that the hands are on the ground and the head bowing to the earth.

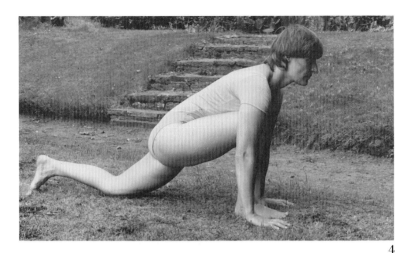

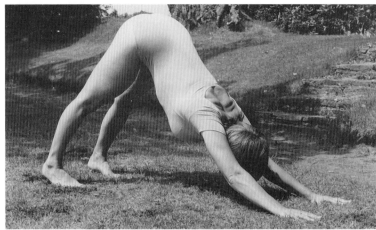

4

6

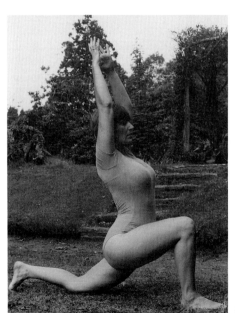

5

Inhale, lift your head and chest, exhale, stretch the left leg out and back to bring the foot as far back behind as you can. Bending the knee, allow the right buttock to come down while you keep the left leg fully extended, the left heel still stretching away for a moment; then let the left knee come lightly down onto the ground (photo 4). Keeping the base of the spine dropped down to stretch the thighs and hips, inhale, lift the chest up and stretch your arms to the side; exhale, take your arms overhead and stretch back, lifting the heart to the sun again and looking up (photo 5). Then inhale; as you exhale, take the hands back down either side of the right foot (photo 4); straighten the left leg, extending it back to lift the hips; exhale, and take the right leg back in line with the left leg to come back into the Face-down Dog pose (photo 6). Stretch into that for a moment, and then on an exhalation go forward into the Face-up Dog pose (photo 7), lifting the heart to the sun again (photo 8). When ready, exhaling, go back into the Face-down Dog pose, bowing down to the earth again (photo 6).

Inhaling, lift your head, and as you exhale take the left leg forward between your hands, drop the base of the spine down and

—151—

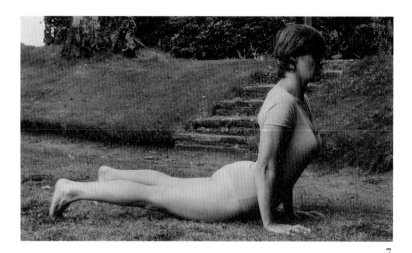

7

Repeat an even number of times, as many as you wish, alternating the leg you move first. You will find you can move into the posture more freely each time because the body loosens up and opens out. Do not continue, though, if you feel exhausted or heavy. The standing poses can be added into the sequence if you wish: move from the Face-down Dog pose into the standing postures by taking one foot forward between the hands, then turning the back leg and hip up to the ceiling so that you are now in a standing pose.

The standing poses are included in the sequence in this way on my Third Yoga Practice Tape, 'Salute to the Sun'.

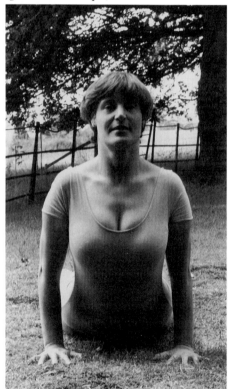

8

with the right heel still stretching away, bring the right knee lightly down onto the ground (as in photo 4, but with the leg positions now reversed). Lift your head and chest up to the sun. Inhaling, stretch your arms to the side; exhaling, take the arms overhead. Stretch the spine up and back, looking up with the head and heart (as in photo 5). Exhale, take the hands down by the left foot; inhale, step firmly on the left foot to bring the right foot forward by the left into *uttanasana* (Standing Forward Bend), photo 3. Let the crown of the head stretch down to the earth and the spine lengthen for a moment. Inhale, lift your head, arms and chest; exhale, come right up to *tadasana* (Mountain pose), arms over the head. Inhale, stretch up out of the hips, exhale, arch the spine backwards, lifting the heart to the sun, opening out a little more to the rising sun (photo 2). Inhaling, return to upright, and exhaling, bring the hands into *namaste* (photo 1).

Take a few easy breaths, feeling the life flowing through you, and lightness in the heart, then repeat the sequence, this time taking the right leg backwards first from *uttanasana* and bringing the right leg forward first when you come out of Face-down Dog pose later in the sequence.

POINTS TO WATCH AND WORK ON

1. When standing and bending backwards (photo 2), keep the lift of your upper back as though you are lifting up and over a bar, and keep extending the heels down into the ground: this will avoid collapsing into the small of the back and straining it.

2. If it is a strain on the lower back to go into and come up out of *uttanasana*, bend the knees as you go down and up.

3. If you have difficulty in bringing the foot right between the hands when stepping forward from the Face-down Dog pose, lift the base of the spine and hips as you step the foot forward to give more space and lightness to the pose.

4. If the shoulders feel tight and uncomfortable in the Dog pose, stretch the hands more down and out to the ground, spreading the whole palm and fingers on the ground (see also the detailed instructions on the two Dog poses).

EFFECTS

In addition to all the benefits of the Face-down and Face-up Dog poses already given, this sequence stimulates and revives the whole system, helps the blood to circulate freely, brings full elasticity and mobility to the hips and legs, relieves congestion, and gives the joy of freedom of movement and a feeling of oneness with all life, above and on the earth.

CHAPTER ELEVEN

Twisting Postures

We do not want our earthly brethren to have their heads in clouds, we want them to have their heads in the sunlight. It does not render a man impractical to live in this way. On the contrary, it makes him more efficient, with all his senses bright, and gives him clarity of thought. Keep your head in the sunlight, and your feet upon beloved Mother Earth, walking the green carpet of earth, so soft and springy, which is comforting, which is homely.

White Eagle, THE WAY OF THE SUN

POSTURES WHICH TWIST the spine laterally around on its axis are important in aligning the energy that flows up and down the spine on all levels. At a physical level they strengthen and tone the small muscles that link one vertebra to the next. No other form of movement in yoga strengthens these muscles in the same way, to prevent the vertebrae closing down on one another. Bad posture causes a contraction of the whole spine as these muscles weaken, so that people actually become shorter as they grow older. Twists prevent such a contraction and the closing down of the vertebrae. At an inner level, practice of the twists allows free movement of the subtle energies that flow from one side of the body to the other and from the base of the spine to the crown of the head. This free-flowing energy is vital to the health and well-being of the spine and therefore of the whole body, inwardly and outwardly.

The extending and spiralling of the energies from the base to the crown has the effect of heightening the perceptions. Thus the mind becomes very alert, increasing our awareness of what is going on in our subconscious and also in others and in the world around us. This helps us to be more sensitive to other people's needs, as well as to our own inner needs, and to be more in tune with nature, becoming one with the energies of nature and the planet as a whole. Such an increase of alertness and awareness brings a much greater ability to concentrate, which is the first stage of meditation.

However, it is very important to stretch and extend the spine before twisting, so these postures are always practised towards the end of a sequence. Stretch the spine well in standing postures, Dog poses, or forward bends to begin with. Twists generally follow back bends in a yoga session as they correct any strain in the spine caused by incorrect practice of the back bends or uneven movement in the hip-joints.

Twists are always practised to the right first, as the movement then goes with the internal flow of energy from the liver (on the right) clockwise around the body to the spleen (on the left). The spleen is responsible for eliminating toxins from the system, so movement on the right first and then on the left helps this elimination and cleanses the whole system.

Be aware of the life and extension that these postures bring to the spine, and the resultant alertness and tuning-up of the mind. Do not let the mind lead, but let the movement come from the base of the spine and spiral all the way up the spine to the head and back down again so that there is a balancing of the energies along the spine.

Bharadvajasana I (Mermaid Pose)

Bharadvaja was a great warrior, the father of Drona, who fought the great war in the ancient yogic text, the Mahabharata, of which the Bhagavad Gita is part. All twisting postures are named after warriors, sages and leaders, indicating the level of courage, determination and intelligence that the practice of them brings. This particular pose is also sometimes called the Mermaid because it resembles the shape of a mermaid sitting, and it can be practised in a much gentler, softer way by not turning the head so much.

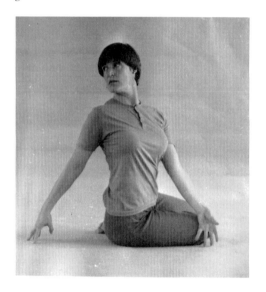

Sit back on the heels. Then take the buttocks to the right of the feet, so that the right buttock is on the ground, the left buttock easing towards the ground, left foot in *virasana* (Hero pose) and knees facing straight forward. Let the left ankle rest on top of the right instep (illustrated opposite, above left). Stretch the spine upwards on an inhalation; on an exhalation turn to the right, taking the right hand onto the ground behind, the left hand against the right thigh as you turn (main photo). Inhale as you stretch up again, exhale as you twist a little more, levering the left hand against the right leg, rotating both shoulders outwards so that the chest opens and lifts. Stay there for a few breaths, continuing to extend the spine, and spiral it upwards and around to the right. Exhale to come forwards and repeat the pose to the left. After some practice the right hand can go behind the back

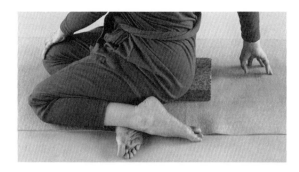

and take hold of the left upper arm, when you are moving to the right (photo, above right). This opens the chest more, but do not go into this further stage if the spine collapses down.

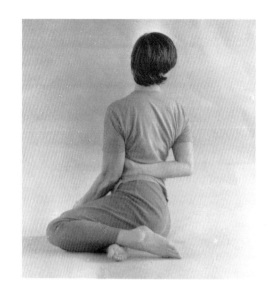

POINTS TO WATCH AND WORK ON

1. If you feel awkward and as though you are collapsing into the right hip (as you turn to the right), put a block under the right buttock: this enables the spine to stretch upwards more. If the knees are uncomfortable, it will also ease them if you do this.

2. IMPORTANT. Do not let the head go ahead of the chest: that is, do not lead with the head, but rather with the heart. Leading with the head makes the posture a strain and puts strain on the neck, so let the head watch where the heart is and go with it. If the head is making a great effort to twist around to look behind, it is divorced from the body, so there will be no all-round awareness of the body's needs, just an ambition to get into the pose.

EFFECTS

This pose awakens the energies along the whole length of the spine, strengthening the lumbar and the dorsal spine in particular, relieving spinal arthritis. It clears the outer mind and heightens the perceptions.

Marichyasana III

This pose is dedicated to Marichi, a great sage, son of the Creator, Brahma, thus indicating that the posture brings wisdom. It follows from *marichyasana I* (given in chapter 10, the forward-bending postures). (*Marichyasana II*, not included in this book, is more difficult for the western body as it involves the Half Lotus posture.)

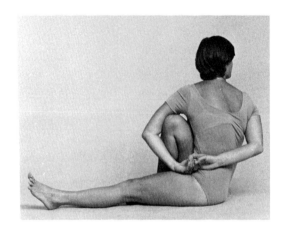

From *dandasana* (Staff pose), bend the right knee up to place the right foot close to the right buttock; stretch the spine up against the right thigh. Take the right hand to the ground behind, the left hand around the right knee (top left-hand photo, opposite). Inhale, stretch the spine up, then exhale as you turn from the base of the spine around to the right, keeping the head relaxed and in line with the chest. Then take the left elbow to the outside of the right knee (lower left-hand photo). Stretch the right foot firmly into the ground and the left heel firmly away, toes pointing to the ceiling. Levering the arm against the leg allows the spine to twist a little more to the right, but do not force or strain the shoulders; rather, concentrate on stretching up, lifting and opening the chest. Stay in the posture as long as you can go on moving and stretching into it and extending the spine. Exhale to come out. Repeat on the left side.

After some time of practising this first stage of the pose, you can stretch the arm out, taking the hand to the other side of the straight leg (right-hand photo), and then go on to the third stage (see main photo, above), taking the left arm—when twisting to the right—around the right knee to take hold of the right hand behind the back. However, do not be in a hurry to get on to these stages; it is more important that the spine can go on lengthening and extending as it twists. So if you feel collapsed down in the chest or waist, go back to the early stages as they give more extension in the first few years of practice.

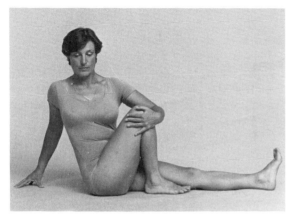

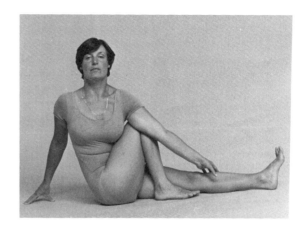

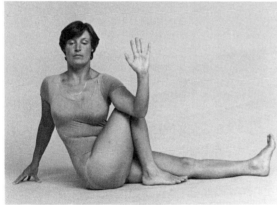

POINTS TO WATCH AND WORK ON

1. If the lumbar spine feels as though it curves back, sit on a block or two, as this lifts the spine up out of the base and hips much more, giving more of a twist to the lower spine.

2. Do not let the bent leg be pushed over the straight leg by the arm, as this just curves the spine: stretch the foot of the bent leg firmly down into the ground to keep the leg firm.

EFFECTS

This pose corrects spinal troubles and relieves pain, so long as the spine is well stretched beforehand. It tones up the liver, spleen and intestines, so relieving sluggishness. It frees tight shoulders and brings alertness to the mind.

Ardha Matsyendrasana I ('Lord of the Fishes' Pose)

Matsyendra is the Lord of the Fishes, responsible for spreading the knowledge of yoga: this *asana* is dedicated to him. When practising the twists after standing postures or forward bends, they are best practised in the order given, so that this one comes last. However, when practising after back bends, start with this one as the spine is more able to stretch up and any unevenness in the hips is corrected in this posture; then follow with *marichyasana III*, and then *bharadvajasana I* (Mermaid pose).

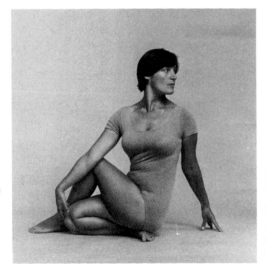

Sit back on the heels; bring the right leg around to place the right foot on the outside of the left knee. Then turn the left heel away so that you sit down across the instep of the left foot, both buttocks being on the left foot, not on the floor (see Points to Watch, no. 1 and the photo, far right). Take the right hand to the ground behind you; take the left hand to the other side of the right knee (top left-hand photo, opposite). Turn from deep in the left hip around to the right. Keeping the upward stretch of the spine, take the left elbow against the outside of the right knee to twist a little further to the right (lower left-hand photo). Inhale as the spine ascends; exhale to twist to the right, remembering to let the heart lead, the head staying in line with the heart. Then repeat on the left side. After practising

this posture for some time you can go on to the position shown in the photo on this page, stretching the arm down to take hold of the opposite knee. However, if this makes the spine curve and collapses the chest, go back to the position shown in the first two photos for some time longer.

POINTS TO WATCH AND WORK ON

1. It is very important to have both buttocks on the foot, as shown in the photo far right: this means the hips and sacrum are even and parallel to the ground rather than at an angle, and then the spine can stretch up straight. It also frees the ankle-joint. However, if this is too uncomfortable on the ankle- and knee-

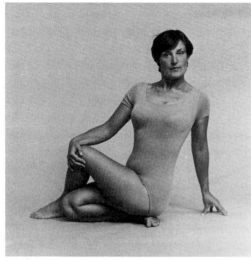

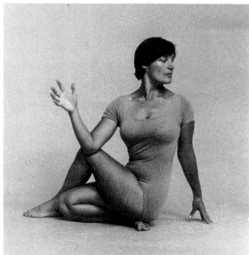

2. If the lower knee is feeling strained, make sure that the knee is straight forward, not pushed to the side by the opposite foot; also stretch the heel that you are sitting on away underneath you: this will relieve the knee.

3. If this posture feels strained and uncomfortable and does not seem to be giving much benefit, then just practise the first two seated twisting postures given here for a while longer, until it feels easier to do this one.

EFFECTS

This posture gives a very good, strong extension and twist of the spine, so all the effects of the other two twisting postures are increased, including the benefits to the lower abdomen, bladder, prostate and ovaries. It lifts us out of the heaviness of the body whilst giving a feeling of being firmly grounded; it allows the spine and the energies around and within the spine to lift and spiral upwards and outwards, so lightening and freeing the spirit.

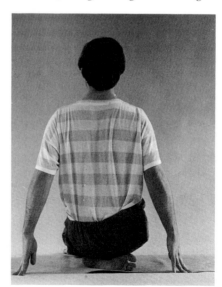

joints, support the right buttock on a block or two for a while until the ankle becomes more flexible.

Jathara Parivartanasana (Lying-down Twist of the Belly)

This gentle, modified version of the classical *jathara parivartanasana* with the knees bent is a very quietening, reviving posture, yet it has a very beneficial massaging effect on all the internal organs and helps to release any strain in the back.

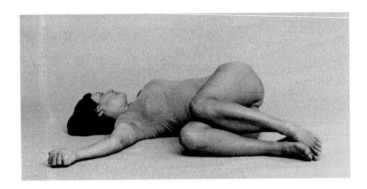

Lie flat on your back; bend your knees up across your chest, hugging them towards you with your arms to stretch the spine out. Roll a little to the left; as you do so ease the right hip away so that you smooth the right side of the lower back out on the floor when you come back to the centre; repeat on the other side.

Then, keeping the knees bent across the chest, spread the arms onto the ground at shoulder level, palms up to the ceiling. Inhale, and as you exhale take the knees out to the left and up towards the left arm to rest on the ground. Then inwardly turn back to the right (if 'inwardly' needs explaining, see chapter 3, pp 54-56). Turn inwardly from the left hip, turn the belly from the left to the right, turn up into the right ribs and the right shoulder and then let the head follow that turn to the right (turn the head last). As you exhale spread the upper back and shoulders on the ground, especially on the right side. Relax there for two to three

minutes (see photo above).

Come back to the centre on an exhalation, then take the knees to the right. Return the knees to the centre; bring your feet onto the floor and relax there for a few moments, feeling the effect of the pose.

POINTS TO WATCH AND WORK ON

1. If there is any strain in the hips or back let the knees rest onto enough cushions or blocks to make it comfortable to stay in the pose.

2. If there is strain in the shoulders or upper arms, bring the arms down a little lower below the level of the shoulders; if that does not relieve the strain put a support (a block or cushion) underneath the arm. Pain in the shoulders means they are moving

and releasing, but do make the pose comfortable enough to be able to relax and let go into it.

3. To stretch and release the lower back a little more, ease and stretch the raised hip and buttock away from you to open out the sacrum and so release the lower back. You may find it helpful to take the left thumb (when the knees are on the left) to the point where the right thigh meets the right hip and ease the hip away from you (see photo in left-hand column).

4. The classical pose is practised with the legs straight and the toes stretching up to meet the hand. After practising for some while with the knees bent, try taking them straight. (It is helpful to do the pose with the knees bent first, then to repeat with them straight.) At first, they may need to bend a little as you go down and come back. The leg-straight position very much intensifies the toning and massaging of the internal organs; Mr Iyengar recommends staying for five to ten minutes on each side to clear away toxins and cleanse the whole system. Gradually build up to this length of time.

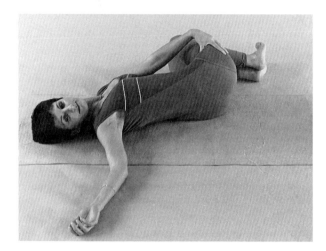

EFFECTS

This posture rests and eases the back, especially after backward and forward bends, and eases out any unevenness in the hips, sacrum and lower back. It releases tension and strain in the upper back and shoulders. It cleanses and tones the liver, spleen, kidneys, stomach, and intestines.

CHAPTER TWELVE

Relaxation and Breathing (*Savasana* and *Pranayama*)

On rising each morning go to your window and stand erect with your mind and heart centred upon God. Do this simply and sincerely, without strain or stress, so that you may soon become attuned to the divine light and learn to know, as surely as the sun rises each day, the true inner meaning of the words, 'Our Father....'. 'I and my Father are One'. Once you contact that Light, you will know that no power on earth or outside the earth can hurt you. Having by your own aspiration drawn within the infinite Light and Power of your Father-Mother God, you are safe within the magical circle of White and Golden Light.

From a White Eagle teaching

THE ATTUNEMENT TO the Divine Light which White Eagle describes provides the essence of *prana*. *Prana* is a very elusive word. Mr Iyengar acknowledges that it is as difficult to explain *prana* as it is to explain God. In LIGHT ON PRANAYAMA he says:

Prana is the energy permeating the universe at all levels.... Prana means breath, respiration, life, vitality, energy or strength...ayama means stretch, extension, expansion, length, breadth, regulation, prolongation, restraint or control. Pranayama thus means the prolongation of breath and its restraint.

We need, when practising *pranayama*, to concentrate on attuning ourselves to the divine life breath. Through our unnatural way of living we have become very out of tune with our breath: we hold our breath, let the breath rush out, strain to take breath in, breathe through our mouths. None of these is natural but we all do them. We need to be able to let go the hold the outer self has

on us, so that we can simply become aware of how the breath naturally comes in and goes out. This sounds as though it should be easy and simple, but we seem to find it extremely difficult to let go the hold we have on ourselves. That is why, in this book, breathing and relaxation have been left until the end. Stretching and working in the postures, if practised without strain, is very releasing as well as giving an openness to the chest, straightening the spine and quietening the mind, so that we are then able to relax and breathe more easily.

Similarly, it should be the easiest thing just to lie down on the ground and relax, but how few of us find it possible to still the body and quieten the mind at will! It comes much more easily after a session of postures than if we just lie down and try to relax: this is because a series of *asanas*, practised in a balanced and effortless way, yet with our full attention, loosens the hold of the outer body so that inner relaxation comes.

AWARENESS AND ATTENTION

Just be aware of letting go the outer physical body in order to let the inner body of light come to life. Let go the hold which the outer mind, the personality, the fears and emotions have on the body and let go, into the earth; trust in the earth, in mother earth.

Savasana (Corpse Pose)

We would say one or two words about relaxation. You are all tense and it is for your good and your health and your peace of mind to consciously practise relaxation. Test yourselves and you will be amazed to discover how tense you are. Now, my children, if you will endeavour to get the feeling that the world is holding you up instead of you holding the world up you will be surprised how much easier you feel. You cannot hold the world up, God does that. And God upholds you, whether you believe it or not—it is true. God is running your life, God is upholding you if you let Him. Now please, dear ones, try to adjust yourselves to the Almighty Power, the Almighty Presence.

From a White Eagle teaching

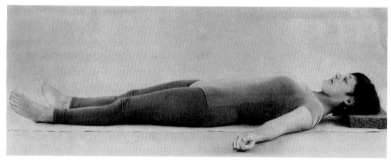

Sava means 'corpse', so in *savasana* we lie absolutely quiet and still without being at all rigid, yet not drifting off to sleep or onto other planes. However, if you do go through a phase of falling asleep in this posture do not worry about it: it just means that you need to sleep at that time. You are probably suffering from a deficit of sleep and the phase will pass when you have caught up on it. Keep the awareness within the physical body and go on letting go, softening and relaxing back into the earth. On some days it will be much easier than on others: sometimes you will be able to relax very easily and quickly and will not need so long, while on other occasions a longer time will be more appropriate. So be patient with yourself; it is very important to be completely comfortable. The photos (see above and overleaf) show variations

of *savasana* to try out, if lying completely flat is not comfortable for you.

It is a good idea to start with the knees bent up to allow the lower back and sacrum to spread out on the ground, and the belly can then relax back into the pelvis. Let the ribs spread out on the ground; let the shoulders relax down away from the ears, and the upper arms release away from the shoulder-joint so that the arms are a little way from the body. Let the throat relax and spread back into the neck. Make sure the neck is quite straight. If it curves backward so that your head drops back, this will constrict the energy-flow down the spine and create a similar curve in the small of the back. It will also stimulate the outer mind and busy thoughts. Put a book or firm block underneath your head: you

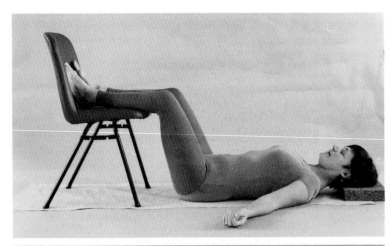

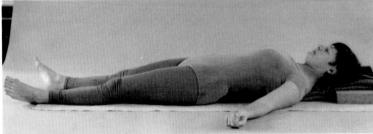

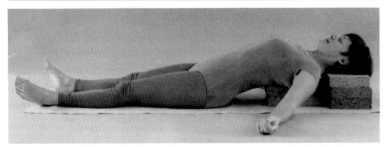

When your back feels relaxed, gently and slowly stretch your legs out one at a time to come into the position shown in the photo on the previous page. Let the thighs release from the hip-joint and let go all the way down to the toes. If this is uncomfortable on your back, put your legs on a chair or stool so that the lumbar spine can stretch out more as illustrated left. If the upper back feels hunched and the shoulders do not feel relaxed, fold a blanket lengthways to about six inches wide and place it under the whole length of the spine (middle photo), or have one or two blocks under the upper back and an extra one under the head (bottom photo, where there are actually *three* blocks under the head and *two* under the shoulders). Once your position is quite comfortable, bring your awareness to your breath without altering the rate of breathing; just go with the exhalation, so that you feel you can relax and let go a little more with each exhalation. If your mind gets busy, your eyes will be looking up towards the mind in the head, the tongue will be pushed up to the roof of the mouth and the facial muscles will have tightened up; so bring the eyes down to the mind in the heart, soften the face, spreading the skin and flesh, and let the tongue spread out in the mouth. Just continue to let go and relax for as long as you feel you need to. Lie in *savasana* for at least five minutes before either getting up or going on to practise *pranayama*.

When you want to come up, gently open your eyes and roll over onto the right side for a few moments, then onto the left side, resting there, then come up to a sitting position from the side. Do not get up quickly: just pause for a moment to bring your hands over your heart in *namaste*, the prayer position, to give thanks for your life and breath.

POINTS TO WATCH

1. If you find it difficult to relax after a series of postures, it is most probably due to the way you are lying, so do alter it. If there is any strain in the lumbar spine, put a block or cushion under

will then be able to feel how the eyes can more easily look down to the chest, so as to concentrate on your breathing and quieten the thoughts.

your knees to relax the lumbar spine or bend your knees up and put your legs on a chair, as shown in the top photo. If your mind is very active, put something under your head, turn the lights out and draw the curtains, or place a cover over your brow and eyes. The little weight of a folded blanket or piece of clothing can do wonders to relax the brain.

2. If you stay too long, you can begin to tense up again and so lose some of the benefits from the postures, so know when you have let go as much as you can and then come up. It is equally important to stay in relaxation long enough really to let go in it, which time will vary from day to day. There is no rule: you need to be aware for yourself.

EFFECTS

Savasana refreshes and rejuvenates the whole body, mind and spirit; it integrates the effects of the *asanas* at all levels of the body. It is in relaxation that we become aware of the effects of the postures that we have just been practising, and so time is needed to allow this to happen. Some of the inner effects that have been given for the *asanas* might not be immediately apparent because this integration takes some time—weeks, months or years—to touch all levels. *Savasana* is very important in bringing the effects through to the inner body, the emotions, the mind and the spirit, so completing the integration.

It replaces lost sleep—twenty minutes of relaxation or meditation is said to be worth four hours of sleep. The practice of yoga itself reduces the amount of sleep needed. Many of us worry a great deal about not having enough sleep; the worry, indeed, prevents us from having a good sleep. Practice of the postures followed by *savasana* helps our sleep pattern greatly and we will very likely find that we do not need as much as we think we do. It is much more beneficial to lie down on the floor in *savasana* in the afternoon than to take a nap in bed, as the whole body and mind can let go of the tensions that seem to make the afternoon nap necessary.

The heart is rested and restored to an easy rhythm by this conscious relaxation: *savasana* is very beneficial for anyone with heart problems, especially ones which prevent them from practising the other postures. It helps to bring down high blood-pressure and reduces any strain on the heart. It also aids the digestive processes.

Ujjayi Pranayama

Ud means 'upward' or 'expanding'. *Jaya* means 'conquest' or 'success'.

This is the basic *pranayama* and gives expansion and lightness to the whole inner and outer body, bringing an ability to control the whole body through the breath, and an ability to concentrate on the breath.

If you have just practised a series of very dynamic postures such as some standing and inverted ones, and Salutations to the Sun, it will not be so easy to practise *pranayama*. It is better practised first thing in the morning before *asana* practice, and followed by meditation; or after quietening postures such as forward bends and seated postures.

Stay in *savasana* as described, giving the body time to relax. If you find it difficult to expand the lungs and chest, this is usually due to bad posture. It helps to lie on a pleated blanket, as shown in the *savasana* photos. Make sure you place yourself quite centrally, with the base of the spine right at the bottom of the blanket or with blocks under the upper back and head. You should feel that the shoulders and ribs can relax down either side of the blanket, to allow the chest and heart to feel open and relaxed. Watch the breath come in and go out. Just observe the rhythm but do not interfere with it. Observe the movement of the belly, ribs, diaphragm and chest. Feel the coolness of the inhalation and the warmth of the exhalation. Breathe always through the nose.

Note how the breath naturally lengthens and deepens even though you are just watching. Feel that you are flowing with the universal breath, that it is almost breathing you. All you have to do is keep your concentration with the breath, do not allow the mind to wander, keep your gaze down. Become aware that the rhythm of the breath is one with the rhythm of the tides and the planets—the breathing-in and breathing-out of the universe—and you feel one with it.

When you feel attuned to the rhythm of the breath, gradually let the exhalation lengthen. Do not let the breath rush out all at once; feel, almost, that you are reluctant to let it go but not straining to hold it at all. Watch the chest lift as you let the breath come in, gently and of its own accord, then keep the lift of the chest on the exhalation, so that the exhalation is slow, gentle and steady. This is not easy, so keep practising. Do not worry if the chest only remains lifted during the exhalation for a little while at first, as it will improve with daily practice.

Feel how the inhalation can gradually lengthen now, spreading the diaphragm and the ribs out gently, without any force or strain; then just let the breath itself decide when to go out and go with it. Feel the natural pause at the end of the exhalation and then let the breath find its way in of its own accord.

If the exhalation apparently wants to rush out uncontrolled, it means you have breathed in too forcefully and quickly, so temper the inhalation a little and the exhalation will feel much better. Conversely, if it feels difficult for the breath to find its way in, it means that you have forcefully pushed the exhalation out, so let the exhalation gently spray out then the inhalation will come more easily.

Mr Iyengar uses an analogy that I find most helpful: he says treat the breath like an old, dear friend. Greet it warmly as it comes in, then feel a little reluctant to let it go: go with it a little way, go with the flow. The inhalation is the drawing-in of the divine life-force, the light; the exhalation is a surrender, a giving-up of the self, of the ego. So feel that surrender, that total giving, on the exhalation; but do not force or strain in any way. Do not make any noise, nor push the breath out or force it in. Just watch and let the breath come in and go out. You need do nothing but concentrate, and the rest will come naturally. Do not continue longer than is reasonable at first, as once the mind wanders it is difficult to bring it back.

After a while of practising this gentle form of breathing you may want to go a little further to look at the difference between the two sides of your body and balance them. To do this just bring your awareness all the way down the length of the left side and let yourself feel the breath come up through the left foot, into the left hip, into the ribs, chest, shoulder and left hemisphere of the brain, and then breathe out through the left side, relaxing the left side a little more out to the side and down into the ground. Do this for several breaths until you feel that you have touched and brought life and awareness to every cell of the left side. Then come back to the centre for a few breaths. Repeat on the right side.

There may be an awareness of great differences between the two sides, and so you may feel the need to stay on one side longer than the other or to come back to the side you started on. It is better to start with the left side, as this is the more intuitive, aware, more feminine side, and connects to the right side of the brain. We tend to have over-developed the left side of our brain (the logical, rational side) in our society, hence the right side of our body is more developed. So let the left side come into its own first, and then work to bring balance. Come back to the centre when you feel that you have brought life and awareness to both sides, and feel now how much easier it is to let the breath come in easily—gently, yet fully—to both sides.

Very gently, when you are quite ready, bring yourself back; do not get up quickly. Roll first to one side, resting there a moment, and then to the other, before sitting up. You can follow into a meditation if you wish to do so, in a seated position.

POINTS TO WATCH

1. If you feel any dizziness or discomfort or coldness afterwards it means that you have tried to take too deep a breath and pushed the air forcefully out—and then probably sat up too quickly. We are so used to forcing a deep breath then pushing it all out to the absolute limit. This is not necessary and causes a lot of strain on the whole system. In fact the breathing, when practised in this gentle, gradual way, brings full extension to the lungs and full interchange of gases in the system in a much more balanced and complete way than forcefully 'trying' to do so.

2. It would be helpful if a friend or relative could read this section to you as though they were a teacher giving instructions, while you relax. Then it is much easier to follow. You may find it helpful to work with my own tape, 'A First Yoga Practice Tape'.

EFFECTS

This gentle, simple breathing soothes and brings control of the nervous system, and quietens and controls the mind. It is very helpful for any condition of anxiety, tension, high blood-pressure or heart disease, headaches, migraine, menstrual problems and lack of energy. It helps us to attune to the Star.

Remember, particularly with the breathing, that it takes some time before we feel we are making any progress and so do not feel tempted to give up. Think of White Eagle's words:

Train yourselves to catch a vision of the Master over the heads of the throng, to hear his voice in your heart, guiding you gently to do those things which you have to do with courage and with peace. Then, my brother, you will not be without joy or hope. If things do not happen as you want them to happen, know that a better way is being found. Trust, and never forget that the true way is the way of love. Flowers do not force their way with great strife. Flowers open to perfection slowly in the sun.

White Eagle, THE QUIET MIND

Meditation

In your meditation we direct you first of all to rise to the apex of the golden triangle and there meditate on the Great White Light or the Golden One, the Christos. As you go directly and earnestly to that point and focus your worship, your adoration, your consciousness in that universal and infinite Light, at the same time bring all your devotion, all your power to that one supreme point. This creates in you the perfectly straight line of light from the base of your spine to the crown of your head, like the mason's plumb line. Not only is your body straight, and the power rising straight up through your body, but all your concentration is on God, on what is good, what is lovely, what is beautiful, what is true, just and wise—the whole being is brought into poise, into straightness.

White Eagle, in THE JEWEL IN THE LOTUS, by Grace Cooke

Please make sure you have read the section on meditation in the introduction before going on to meditation here.

Following the relaxation and *pranayama*, come up to a comfortable sitting position making sure the spine is straight and the knees are relaxed.

If you are sitting cross-legged, sit up on enough blocks or cushions to allow the knees to relax down below the hips. If the knees are too high in the air they will push you backwards, curving the spine. If your back feels weak and as though it cannot maintain the straight position for a length of time, sit back against the wall. *Baddha konasana* (Cobbler pose), done against the wall, is a very good position for meditating. If the knees are painful, try sitting in *virasana* (Hero pose), on a block or two, so that the spine can be stretched up easily.

Once you are comfortably seated, focus your awareness on the extension upward and the straightness of the spine. Feel the lift this gives to the inner body and the heart, and then let go of the outer body, let go of the mind, the very brain, the ears, the shoulders, and the arms right down to the finger-tips. Let go of the hips, the thighs; let any tension go out through the knees and the feet.

Bring your awareness down out of the head-mind into the mind in the heart. Bring your whole attention to the breath, watch it come and go. Having relaxed and practised the *ujjayi pranayama* lying down, you are now in a very good state to meditate and can go straight into it; if, however, you would like to follow the instructions for *ujjayi pranayama*, they transfer perfectly well to a sitting position. If you are going straight into this meditation from daily life, it is helpful to do a little *pranayama* first.

Then just watch your breath, and centre in your heart.

If you would like some guidance on meditation the following sequence is often used in my classes, as it follows on well from *pranayama*.

Feel the breath coming in right from the base as though it comes right up through the earth. Feel that firm base of the earth, as the breath comes and goes, like the broad base of a triangle or pyramid; as you reach the top of the inhalation feel the apex of the pyramid rising up the spine, a little higher at the high point of each subsequent inhalation. As you exhale, keep that awareness on the apex—the high point—so that the inner body, the heart, stays lifted throughout the exhalation, whilst the outer body lets go, spreads to the sides and down a little more.

Be with the breath in this way until the apex of the triangle comes right up through the heart, and then the head, until a point above the head is reached, aspiring upwards. Look down from that point above the head as you exhale, seeing the outer body let go of its hold more and more, keeping that firm base in the hips earthed on the ground. As you visualize this upward-pointing triangle, representing man on earth aspiring upwards, heavenwards, see the downward point of the triangle being drawn down from the heavens to fit perfectly over the upward, aspiring triangle to create the Star. Your heart is the central point of the Star; as the breath gently comes and goes, just be there in that Star, in your heart.

During your meditation, if you like, say any affirmation that would help you (there are many given in the Introduction). When you are ready to finish, bring your hands over your heart in *namaste*, the prayer position, and bow to the earth giving thanks to God and the earth for your life, your breath. Then bow in thanks to those around you, seen and unseen.

This gesture, *namaste*, an Indian greeting, means that when I am in that place in me and you are in that place in you, then you and I are one.

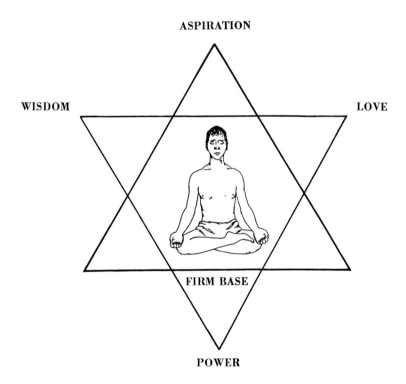

ASPIRATION

WISDOM

LOVE

FIRM BASE

POWER

CHAPTER THIRTEEN

The Practice of Yoga during Pregnancy and After

Your body is the instrument for God's work; through your body comes the power to create bodies for incoming egos. What a sacred work is yours! God will use the gifts which you give Him to glorify the earth. Through your physical body you will be able to work in partnership with God. According to your purity and love of God you will be enabled to attract to the physical body which you can create, those highly evolved souls who are waiting to come into incarnation, to be born into pure bodies that will give them every opportunity in the great work of bringing brotherhood upon earth.

White Eagle, in SUN MEN OF THE AMERICAS, by Grace Cooke

IF THE ESSENCE of yoga is really to be understood and practised, it is important to remember throughout your pregnancy the great privilege and honour of having been chosen to be a mother by the soul of your baby, and always to tune into the needs and desires of the baby in whatever you do during pregnancy. It is also very helpful to remember that the soul coming to you has much to teach you, if you can tune in to it. Your baby is a very evolved, intelligent, sensitive being who is full of the purest love for you, the mother who is carrying it. The bond created during this very special time, between you as mother and your child, will always be there, and creates a firm foundation for his or her time on earth. So consciously communicate to your baby what you are doing and why you are doing it and be awake to the response you get from them—so that you intuitively know what is best for both of you. You will understand how it is possible to do this as you try to do it.

It is advisable to have an experienced teacher during pregnancy and afterwards, one who has practised yoga during pregnancy herself, or who has experience of the practice of yoga by others during pregnancy. You may like to work with my own tape,

'Yoga in Pregnancy'. However, here are some basic rules to be followed.

If you were practising yoga before you became pregnant, then as long as it feels comfortable to do so you can go on doing those postures which you were happy with beforehand, with the exception of *Surya Namaskar* (Salutation to the Sun), arm balances (postures which take all the weight on the arms, although some women are happy still doing *adho mukha vrksasana*—Full Arm-balance—if helped up and down) and twists that restrict the baby in any way, such as *marichyasana III. Bharadvajasana I* (Mermaid pose) is a suitable alternative. In earlier pregnancy lying on the belly with a blanket folded under the pubis is fine, but as soon as this feels uncomfortable, stop doing it. It is not a time to start any new postures. However, many people who have never done yoga before actually start during pregnancy, as it has been found greatly to help labour and birth pains. It is necessary to go very gently and slowly. Look for a class, if you can: some teachers, including myself, run special classes.

If the hormonal adjustment to pregnancy in the first three months is not easy, if there is nausea, tiredness and discomfort, then it is better not to do any *asanas* for those three months. There is also a risk of miscarriage at this time if care is not exercised. Just rest in the relaxation pose *savasana* (Corpse pose), and practise some gentle *pranayama*, directing the energy around the womb to help the adjustment. Recommence the *asanas* when your body has adjusted and you feel like moving again. Always be guided by how your body feels: you will be more centred in and aware of your body during pregnancy than you were before. There are some women who just need to do *savasana* for nine months, and there are others who can carry on doing

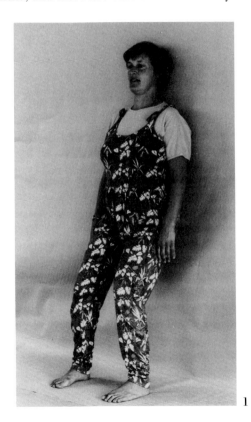

1

everything they did before with no difficulty right up to the moment of birth. Some will not want to do any postures at all for certain stages of the pregnancy. Tune into your needs and the baby's. Just do a few standing poses if you like, so long as you do not become tired in them; or you may prefer to leave them out almost completely, as I did. I had practised standing postures regularly for many years before becoming pregnant and when pregnant I felt very much that my body needed a complete rest from them apart from *tadasana* (Mountain pose) and *vrksasana* (Tree pose). My body had become very strong through practising standing postures and needed to soften up during pregnancy. So again, tune into what your body and your baby needs—you may need more strengthening at this time.

The photos in this chapter were taken at the end of the sixth month of my pregnancy.

If you get backache and the lumbar spine feels very curved as your centre of gravity is taken forward by the position of the baby, then it is very helpful to practise *tadasana* against the wall (as shown in photo 1) and with the knees a little bent at first, so that the small of the back can relax back into the wall, with the upper back and head resting against it. Tilt the top rim of the pelvis (the iliac crest) up and back—away from the pubis—so that the baby relaxes back in the pelvis. When that feels comfortable then gently stretch the legs by extending the heels into the ground and the buttock-bones up the wall. Do not push the knees back. It is better to have the legs a little bent rather than locked back in the knees, as locked-back knees have the effect of pushing the small of the back forward into an uncomfortable arch again.

Then come away from the wall and, exhaling, go forward into *uttanasana* (Standing Forward Bend) onto a chair (as shown in photo 2, overleaf) with the legs a little bent as you go forward. Then lift up the buttock-bones as you flatten and straighten the back, so that the legs stretch but do not lock back. Soften the belly and give the baby room to spread. This opening and relaxing of the belly area is very important in all the postures in order

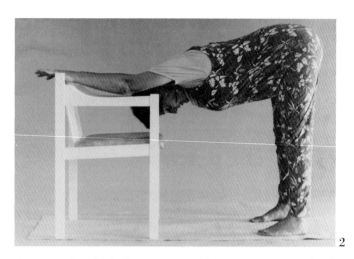

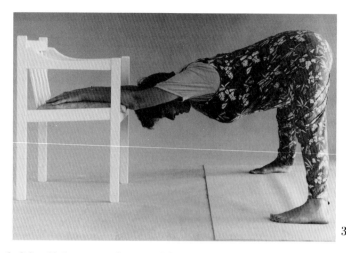

to make space for the baby to move and grow: never restrict the belly at all in the postures. Come up by bending the knees a little and lifting from the pelvis, exhaling. Then take the legs wide into *prasarita padottanasana* (Wide Leg-stretch Forward Bend, photo 3) and repeat the instructions to stretch forward, a little lower this time, onto the seat of the chair.

If after the practice of these three postures you feel like doing a few more standing postures, go on to *vrksasana* (Tree pose); then *utthita trikonasana* (Triangle pose) against the wall; *utthita parsvakonasana* (Stretched-flank pose), also against a wall; and if you are able to balance, *ardha chandrasana* (Half Moon pose) against a wall with a low stool to put your hand on. Instructions for all of these are given in chapter 5 (standing postures). They all move and open the pelvis, the sacrum and the ileum which help greatly in labour as long as they are not practised too strongly and forcefully.

Squatting (*malasana*, the Garland pose) is also very freeing on the sacrum and the pelvic-floor muscles (as shown in photos 4 and 5). This is a traditional way of giving birth, as just the position itself opens the vagina and helps the passage of the baby. If the

heels lift off the ground, put a block under them for support, as shown in photo 5.

Then sit in *virasana* (Hero pose)—always use as much support as you need to make the posture comfortable to relax into. So when you lie back in *supta virasana* (as shown in photo 6) have as much support as is needed so that there is no strain on the back and the belly can soften and relax back into the pelvis, giving space for the baby. Do not go so far down that it is a strain to get out of the pose again. When you come up, sit on your heels, and take your knees wide apart. Exhaling, go forwards and take your head to the ground. For full instructions on these postures refer to chapter 9.

In *parvatasana* (Cross-legged Forward Bend, in the upright position, see pages 95-96) twist first to the right and then to the left; and then go forward a little way over a chair (which you need to have ready beforehand), relaxing your brow down onto it. Let the belly (and baby!) spread down between your legs; relax there for a few minutes. In forward bends such as *janu sirsasana* (Forward Bend over each Leg) do not go forwards but stretch up with a belt, as shown in photo 7. When the left leg is bent, take

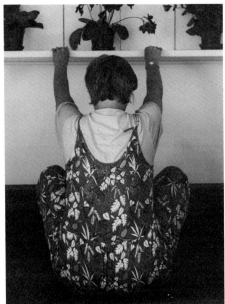

4

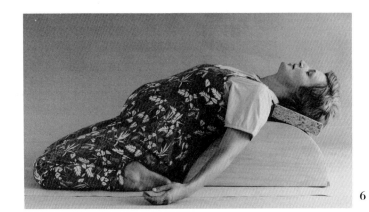

6

hold of the belt with the left hand and take the right hand behind, so that you are turning the belly out of the left hip towards the right, stretching the spine up, and then bring the right hand forward to take hold of the belt, keeping the spine stretched up. Come out of it exhaling and change to the other side.

In *upavistha konasana* (Seated Angle pose) lean back a little

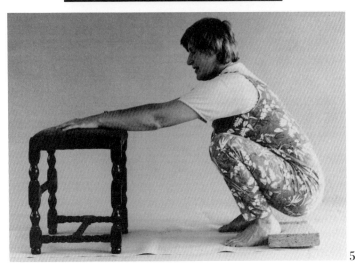

5

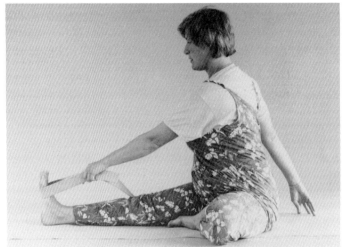

7

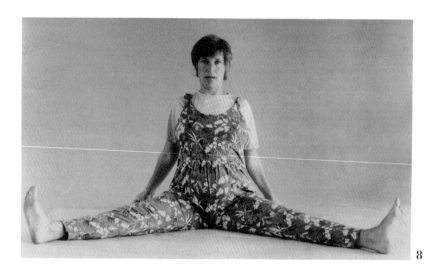

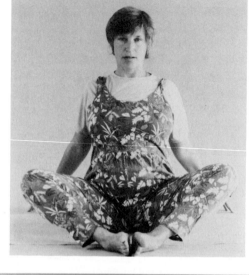

8

9

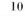

10

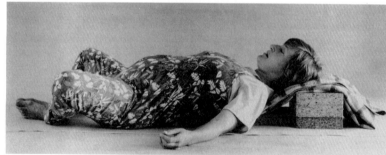

on your hands (photo 8) so that again you make space for the baby. Do the same in *baddha konasana* (Cobbler pose, photo 9), sitting on a block if necessary. It is useful to practise *baddha konasana* against a wall, thus enabling the sacrum and pelvic muscles to let go, so that you can stay there comfortably for a while—it is a good posture for meditation. Also practise *supta baddha konasana* with support under the head and upper back as shown (Cobbler pose lying on the floor, photo 10). The best twist to practise is *bharadvajasana I* (Mermaid pose). Follow the instructions given in chapter 11 (twisting postures); it will often be best to sit on a block. This pose strengthens and lengthens the spine, relieving backache without in any way closing the belly, as the other twists would.

Inverted poses are very beneficial during pregnancy as they relieve heaviness and pressure downwards, and tiredness. They also prevent varicose veins and oedema (swelling due to water retention) developing, both of which are common in pregnancy. However if you did not start practising them before you were pregnant this is not the time to start. Rather, just put your legs up the wall as shown in photos 11 and 12. These will give a gentler, more modified effect with similar benefits.

It is fine to practise *sirsasana* (Head-stand, photo 13) during pregnancy, as long as you practised it before you were pregnant and your blood pressure is not high. Later on in pregnancy have someone to help you up and down into it so that it is not a jolt on the baby. Babies usually love being turned upside-down in the

—176—

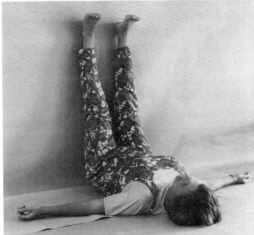

11

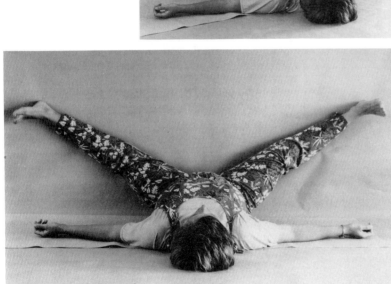

12

13

womb—it gives them freedom of movement; I could always feel mine enjoying it. Refer to chapter 8 (inverted postures) for full instructions .

Salamba sarvangasana (Shoulder-stand) needs to follow the Head-stand. Go straight into the modified form of the Shoulder-stand, using the wall, with blocks underneath your back—known as *viparita karani*—photo 14. Have two or three blocks ready by your side and take yourself close to the wall with the legs up the wall, back flat on the floor, buttocks touching the wall. Relax there for a few minutes. Then bend your knees and take your feet flat onto the wall. Inhale, and spread your feet into the wall. Exhale, and lift your lower back and pelvis up off the ground and slide the blocks underneath your pelvis. Make sure

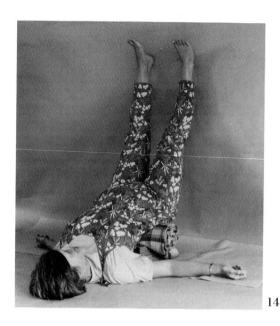

15

16

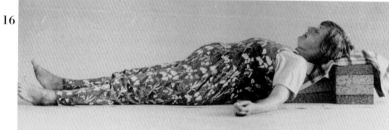

14

your buttocks are just off the blocks as it will then be more comfortable on your back; try two blocks and if you do not feel enough lift put a third one underneath. Then stretch your legs up the wall. It needs to be comfortable enough to stay there for five to ten minutes. If it is not, adjust the position of the blocks. If there is any pressure in your head or tightness in your throat, then come off the blocks and lie with the back flat on the ground. In either position, relax your pelvis down into the ground and let the baby relax back in the pelvis. If you want to go over into *supta konasana* (Wide-angled Plough pose, photo 15), place two chairs or stools wide apart so that one foot can rest on one stool and the other on the other one. Make sure you lift the buttock-bones up to stretch the spine. Stay as long as is comfortable—if there is any pressure on the head or the belly then come down. Finish always with the relaxation pose *savasana* (Corpse pose), but do not lie absolutely flat as this can restrict the blood and

oxygen supply to the baby. You will gradually need more and more support under the head and upper back (as shown in photo 16). Use blocks, folded blankets, pillows or cushions. Many women need to be almost sitting in the final stages of pregnancy. Whilst there, practise the *ujjayi pranayama* given in chapter 12 (relaxation and breathing). It is the breathing recommended by the French obstetrician Frédéric Leboyer in his book THE ART OF BREATHING. It will be of immense help during labour and will greatly help you to overcome any fear and tension beforehand; and it can be used during labour to regulate, quieten and calm the breath and the whole system.

Always remember that your body, even at rest, is working harder than a mountaineer's. All the vital organs are doing an enormous amount of extra work in order first to build the baby's life-support system and then nourish it and excrete its waste. So do not push yourself to the point of tiredness either in your yoga practice or in your daily life. Although I had previously practised a great many *asanas* daily, I found that I wanted to do much more relaxation, *pranayama* and meditation in preparation for my baby's arrival into this world, and also to contact the soul and heart of the little life growing inside me. I also felt very much inspired to chant during meditation, and subsequently read in Leboyer's book that chanting and singing are very helpful in control of the breathing in labour and in the control of the labour itself.

Take it especially easily in the last month of pregnancy, only doing what feels right for you without much effort being involved. Rest, relaxation and meditation are most important at this time to lead you up to and prepare you for a most important event in your life, so that you are relaxed and calm when it is your baby's time to come into the world.

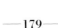

After Pregnancy

The yogic system gives advice on the post-natal phase that is rather different from that given by modern medicine. Yoga works on the principle that there is an enormous internal adjustment needed, on an energy level, a hormonal level (the hormones directly connect to the energy centres), a psychological and emotional level, and a spiritual level too, in the first three months of pregnancy and in the first three months after the birth of the baby.

During these times we need to be very gentle and caring towards ourselves, as does our partner and those close to us, and allow nature to make this adjustment without imposition from the outside. The forceful exercises given by doctors for the time immediately after birth seem to me a gross imposition on a delicately-balanced, highly-sensitized woman, and I have yet to meet a woman who felt that they were what she wanted to do at that time. They seem to have been developed out of a masculine-dominated system that feels the need to *do*, to force the will, to strain and push.

Yoga advocates that you do nothing apart from relaxation and meditation, but instead allow the adjustment to take place and simply care for your baby for the first two or three months after the birth (at least three months, if there was any tearing in the vagina and you needed stitches, or you had a caesarian section). Meditation is particularly helpful during and after pregnancy to help the adjustment in yourself, to help the incoming soul and to tune into the wonder of life, birth and death. Allow yourself to just be. Give up *doing* for a while—it will not be for ever—and just enjoy being. Feel the honour, the great privilege of being a vehicle for a new life, the incarnation of a soul coming to clothe itself in a body to develop and learn alongside you. Tune into the baby in your meditation, talk to it, reassure it, communicate with him or her on a heart-to-heart level. This will greatly help the transition of that soul into a body, which is not an easy transition, and one that twentieth-century attitudes make even more difficult, although they are slowly changing now.

Once you start again, take your body gently and easily into the postures without any strain, being mindful of the tremendous changes that have gone on in your body, and awakening to the vitality, health and well-being that the practice of yoga naturally gives.

CHAPTER FOURTEEN

Healing your Body, Mind and Emotions

We suggest that those who suffer—particularly because of blindness or defective vision—may have come to the last step upon a road of soul-cleansing or development. We are too apt to say, 'so and so is suffering as a result of karma'. This term is used a little loosely. Perhaps it would be more correct to say, 'so and so's body is suffering because he, the soul, has reached the end of a certain path of growth or learning which has been undertaken'.

White Eagle, THE LIVING WORD OF ST JOHN

Yoga for the Physically Handicapped

A WHOLE BOOK could be written on this subject and it could be that many people who are handicapped will find the actual postures in this book off-putting, because they appear to be too difficult. However, there is much that can be done through yoga. Do look for a teacher, for there are many who run special classes and many who are willing to come to your home to give personal help. The philosophy, meditation and affirmations are a great help when bodily movement is inhibited.

Even if you cannot do a complete posture, read all the instructions, to give yourself the awareness of the body the posture brings. For example, the instructions for *tadasana* (Mountain pose) can be followed standing against a wall with sticks or sitting in a wheelchair. The *savasana* (Corpse pose) and *pranayama* can be done sitting in an armchair or lying on the bed. The meditation can be done anywhere. You may be able gradually to do some of the others with help and support from chairs, walls, sticks and/or a friend. The awareness given just by connecting the mind to the body in the detail of the posture, even if you cannot move very far into it, has been found to be very helpful in degenerative diseases such as multiple sclerosis, motor neurone disease and muscular dystrophy.

Special help can be given at the main centres of the White Eagle Lodge, while the Yoga for Health Foundation at Ickwell Bury, Bedfordshire, specifically caters for the handicapped. A book by Barbara Brosnan called YOGA FOR THE HANDICAPPED is very helpful and informative.

The deep underlying principles of yoga would state that your Higher Self has chosen this condition for your spirit to grow and evolve, and also to teach those around you to love. There is evidence of tremendous love in handicapped children particularly—they emanate love and teach those around them to love at the deepest level. So acceptance here is very important without giving up; just letting go the deeply-held hurt and doing what you are able to for yourself.

Postures, Relaxation and Meditation to Practise for Certain Disorders

A

Abdominal pain and cramps: all twists especially *jathara parivartanasana* (Lying-down Twist of the Belly), *paschimottanasana* (Sitting Forward Bend). Relaxation—*savasana* (Corpse pose) with legs on a chair.

Acne: *salamba sarvangasana* (Shoulder-stand) held for at least four minutes clears toxins out of the system. Do it supported by a wall or chair if you feel it a strain to hold for this long.

Aids: *salamba sirsasana* (Head-stand), *salamba sarvangasana* (Shoulder-stand), *setu bandha sarvangasana* (Bridge pose), *supta virasana, baddha konasana* (Cobbler pose) against the wall, standing postures with back against the wall—just *utthita trikonasana* (Triangle pose) if very weak—*paschimottanasana* (Sitting Forward Bend). Relaxation and meditation, *pranayama*, twists.

Anaemia: inverted poses to stimulate blood, relaxation, *pranayama*, meditation.

Ankles: weakness and strains. Standing postures with the back foot firmly against a wall: *virasana* (Hero pose), with support of a folded blanket underneath the ankles and as many blocks as needed to make it possible to relax there for five minutes. Forward bends with a belt around the foot. Inverted postures to relieve strain and help blood supply to area.

Anorexia: *salamba sarvangasana* (Shoulder-stand), *baddha konasana* (Cobbler pose) against the wall for ten minutes, *supta virasana* for five to ten minutes. Relaxation, *pranayama* and meditation.

Anxiety: *uttanasana* (Standing Forward Bend), *prasarita padottanasana* (Wide Leg-stretch Forward Bend), all sitting forward bends and inverted poses. Meditation.

Apathy: all inverted poses, *Surya Namaskar* (Salutation to the Sun), *baddha konasana* (Cobbler pose).

Appendix problems: all twists especially *jathara parivartanasana* (Lying-down Twist of the Belly), inverted poses especially *salamba sarvangasana* (Shoulder-stand), and *setu bandha sarvangasana* (Bridge pose).

Arms, stiffness, aching, strain, weakness: *adho mukha svanasana* (Face-down Dog pose), *jathara parivartanasana* (Lying-down Twist of the Belly), *adho mukha vrksasana* (Full Arm-balance).

Arthritis:

Spine—standing postures (back flat against the wall) especially *tadasana* (Mountain pose), *utthita trikonasana* (Triangle Pose), *utthita parsvakonasana* (Stretched-flank pose), *adho mukha svanasana* (Face-down Dog pose), *uttanasana* (Standing Forward Bend) with hands on a chair; back bends, especially *urdhva dhanurasana* (Face-up Bow pose or Back Arch) over a chair, *virasana* (Hero pose); twists.

Hips—standing postures (back flat against the wall) especially *tadasana* (Mountain pose), *utthita trikonasana* (Triangle pose), *utthita parsvakonasana* (Stretched-flank pose), supported *virasana* (Hero pose), *baddha konasana* (Cobbler pose) against wall, put blocks under knees for support if hips are painful. *Parvatasana* (Cross-legged Forward Bend), *janu sirsasana* (Forward Bend over each Leg) with block under knee if hips painful, *upavistha konasana* (Seated Angle pose), legs up the wall (first stage of Shoulder-stand, p. 126), *savasana* (Corpse pose) with legs on a chair.

Knees—*tadasana* (Mountain pose), *utthita trikonasana* (Triangle pose), *parsvottanasana*, *utthita parsvakonasana* (Stretched-flank pose) with hand on chair if painful on knee. *Virasana* (Hero pose) (sitting as high as possible without severe pain—there are chairs for sitting in a modified Hero pose). *Baddha konasana* (Cobbler pose), all forward bends, especially *upavistha konasana* (Seated Angle pose).

Shoulders—*salamba sirsasana* (Head-stand) on a chair, *setu bandha sarvangasana* (Bridge pose), twists especially *jathara parivartanasana* (Lying-down Twist of the Belly), and *bharadvajasana I* (Mermaid pose).

Fingers and wrists—*svanasana* (Face-up and Face-down Dog Poses), *parsvottanasana*.

Asthma: *tadasana* (Mountain pose), *vrksasana* (Tree pose), *utthita trikonasana* (Triangle Pose), *utthita parsvakonasana* (Stretched-flank pose), *parsvottanasana*, *supta virasana* with blocks under upper back to open chest out. All back bends especially *setu bandha sarvangasana* (Bridge pose) over a stool, with back over a chair relaxing there for five to ten minutes. *Supta baddha konasana* (Cobbler pose done lying down) and *baddha konasana* against wall with block or folded blanket behind upper back to open chest out. *Bharadvajasana I* (Mermaid pose). Relaxation with blanket or block under upper back (as illustrated in the photo on p. 166); *ujjayi pranayama*, meditation on watching the breath.

B

Back Problems:
Base of Spine—*supta virasana*, *uttanasana* (Standing Forward Bend) and *parsvottanasana* with hands on chair, *urdhva mukha svanasana* (Face-down Dog pose), *Surya Namaskar* (Salutation to the Sun), *dandasana* (Staff pose), *upavistha konasana* (Seated Angle pose), and *baddha konasana* (Cobbler pose) on a lift (block or folded blanket).

Lumbar Spine (small of back)—all standing postures (if back aches with back flat against the wall) especially *utthita* and *parivrtta trikonasana* (Triangle and Reverse Triangle poses). Back bends supported with chair or stool at first, forward bends with a belt stretching up as illustrated (do not go forwards), twists especially *ardha matsyendrasana I* ('Lord of the Fishes' pose). Relaxation—*savasana* (Corpse pose) with legs on a chair.

Dorsal spine (upper back)—all standing postures especially *ardha chandrasana* (Half Moon pose), back flat against the wall at first; all back bends; all twists concentrating on opening chest out, *supta virasana*. Relaxation with blocks or blanket under upper back (photo, p. 166)

Balance problems: all standing poses especially *tadasana* (Mountain pose), *utthita trikonasana* (Triangle pose), *vrkasana* (Tree pose), *ardha chandrasana* (Half Moon pose), *salamba sirsasana* (Head-stand) (after practising standing postures for a year at least).

Bladder problems: all back bends and twists especially *jathara parivartanasana* (Lying-down Twist of the Belly).

Blood Pressure:
High—forward bends (resting head on blocks or cushion placed on top of legs or on a chair placed over legs). Relaxation, meditation.

Low—short stay Head-stand or Shoulder-stand (keeping head down on the ground for five minutes after coming down to prevent dizziness). Relaxation, meditation.

Bowel disorders: all standing poses especially reverse ones after stretched version; all twists, especially *jathara parivartanasana* (Lying-down Twist of the Belly) and *marichyasana III*; inverted poses for a short time.

Bronchitis: *salamba sirsasana* (Head-stand), *salamba sarvangasana* (Shoulder-stand) supported, using wall and blocks under hips to open chest or over a chair (stay in it for five to ten minutes). *Setu bandha sarvangasana* (Bridge pose) supported on a low stool or several blocks, for five to ten minutes. *Ujjayi pranayama* and relaxation, upper back and head lifted on blocks.

C

Cancer: great variation according to stage and where it is; concentrate on meditation and *pranayama*, visualizing healthy cells being drawn in on inhalation and unhealthy ones going out on exhalation.

If in internal organs, or leukaemia—*salamba sirsasana* (Head-stand) and *salamba sarvangasana* (Shoulder-stand), *svanasana* (Face-down Dog pose) where possible, *supta virasana, setu bandha sarvangasana* (Bridge pose).

If in spine—relaxation and *svanasana* (Face-down Dog pose) (see under Hodgkin's disease).

Cholesterol (high): inverted poses, *Surya Namaskar* (Salutation to the Sun) do not allow pressure in the head to build up—make sure breathing is easy; *supta virasana, setu bandha sarvangasana* (Bridge pose). Relaxation, *pranayama*.

Colds: *tadasana* (Mountain pose), *trikonasana* (Triangle pose), inverted poses, forward bends, *supta virasana*. Relaxation.

Conjunctivitis: *salamba sarvangasana* (Shoulder-stand), *setu bandha sarvangasana* (Bridge pose); forward bends.

Constipation: inverted poses; standing poses; twists. Relaxation—concentrating on letting go, especially the internal organs.

D

Deafness: inverted poses, *svanasana* (Face-up and Face-down Dog poses).

Depression: back bends—several times for ten minutes, building up to twenty minutes; *uttanasana* (Standing Forward Bend) *supta virasana, salamba sirsasana* (Head-stand), *salamba sarvangasana* (Shoulder-stand). Meditation on light.

Diarrhoea: forward bends, *salamba sarvangasana* (Shoulder-stand).

Dizziness: *paschimottanasana* (Sitting Forward Bend) with head resting on a block or a cushion.

E

Emphysema: supported *supta virasana, salamba sarvangasana* (Shoulder-stand). *Pranayama*, relaxation.

Epilepsy: (under guidance of a teacher) *salamba sarvangasana* (Shoulder-stand), *halasana* (Plough pose), *paschimottanasana* (Sitting Forward Bend). Relaxation, breathing and meditation.

Eyes, long and short sight: *salamba sirsasana* (Head-stand), *salamba sarvangasana* (Shoulder-stand), *uttanasana* (Standing Forward Bend), *paschimottanasana* (Sitting Forward Bend). Practise looking into the distance a moment then close-up four times, then cup hands over eyes, closing eyes for one minute. Repeat three times, then meditate.

Cataracts and glaucoma: follow the above but take care in *sirsasana*—use a chair under the guidance of a teacher.

See also Conjunctivitis.

F

Fever: relaxation, *pranayama*.

Flatulence: inverted poses and twists.

G

Gallstones: *tadasana* (Mountain pose), *utthita* and *parivrtta trikonasana* (Triangle and Reverse Triangle poses), *utthita parsvakonasana* (Stretched-flank pose), *parsvottanasana, janu* *sirsasana* (Forward Bend over each Leg), *ardha baddha padma paschimottanasana* (Half-Lotus Forward Bend); all back bends and inverted poses.

Genital Problems: all standing poses, concentrating on lifting the pelvis up off the thighs, the top rim of the pelvis moving back; twists; *supta virasana* .

Glandular problems: *salamba sarvangasana* (Shoulder-stand), *setu bandha sarvangasana* (Bridge pose), *supta virasana, paschimottanasana* (Sitting Forward Bend), relaxation and meditation.

H

Haemorrhoids: standing postures and twists, especially *jathara parivartanasana* (Lying-down Twist of the Belly).

Hay Fever: *tadasana* (Mountain pose), *vrksasana* (Tree pose), *uttanasana* (Standing Forward Bend), *prasarita padottanasana* (Wide Leg-stretch Forward Bend), *supta virasana, salamba sarvangasana* (Shoulder-stand), *setu bandha sarvangasana* (Bridge pose). Relaxation, *pranayama.*

Headaches: *salamba sirsasana* (Head-stand), *adho mukha vrksasana* (Full Arm-balance), *salamba sarvangasana* (Shoulder-stand), *setu bandha sarvangasana* (Bridge pose), all forward bends resting head on a block or cushion placed on top of legs, or on a chair placed over legs. Many headaches are caused by liver and kidney blockages so also follow the postures for those.
See also Migraine.

Heart Problems:
Weakness—all standing postures with back to the wall
Heart attack—relaxation and *pranayama* on a folded blanket (as shown in the photo on p. 166). *Baddha konasana* (Cobbler pose) against the wall. Meditation.
See also Blood pressure.

Heartburn: all standing poses, dog poses and back bends.

Hepatitis: *utthita* and *parivrtta trikonasana* (Triangle and Reverse Triangle poses) (repeat each three times), *utthita* and *parivrtta parsvakonasana* (Stretched-flank and Reverse Stretched-flank Poses), *janu sirsasana* (Forward Bend over each Leg), *ardha baddha padma paschimottanasana* (Half-Lotus Forward Bend), *paschimottanasana* (Sitting Forward Bend); all twists.

Hernia: *tadasana* (Mountain pose), *trikonasana, ustrasana* (Camel pose), keeping front of body relaxed back—do not push the front out; inverted poses; twists. Relaxation, breathing and meditation.

Hip problems, stiffness and pain: all standing postures and all forward bends.

Hodgkin's Disease: *supta virasana*, all back-bends concentrating on opening diaphragm area, and twists.

I

Impotence: inverted poses, back-bends, *Surya Namaskar* (Salutation to the Sun) concentrating on stretching thigh muscles from groin especially in the positionof photo no. 5, p. 151 (one foot and one knee on the ground). Relaxation, *pranayama* and meditation.

Incontinence: *supta virasana, baddha konasana* (Cobbler pose), *upavistha konasana* (Seated Angle pose), *janu sirsasana* (Forward Bend over each Leg), *triang mukhaikapada paschimottanasana* (Forward Bend with one Leg in Hero pose).

Indigestion: *supta virasana, baddha konasana* (Cobbler pose), *siddhasana.* Relaxation.

Influenza: *salamba sirsasana* (Head-stand) briefly, against wall or with help, *salamba sarvangasana* (Shoulder-stand) supported against wall with blocks, or over chair, *setu bandha sarvangasana* (Bridge pose) supported, *supta virasana.*

Insomnia: before retiring—*salamba sarvangasana* (Shoulder-stand) for ten minutes, *halasana* (Plough pose) for five minutes, *paschimottanasana* (Sitting Forward Bend) for five minutes. Relaxation for five minutes.

J

Jaundice: see Liver problems

K

Kidney problems: *utthita* and *parivrtta trikonasana* (Triangle and Reverse Triangle poses), *janu sirsasana* (Forward Bend over each Leg), *paschimottanasana* (Sitting Forward Bend); all twists.

Knee problems: all standing poses, followed by *virasana* (Hero pose), sitting as high as necessary to make the pose comfortable on the knees, *baddha konasana* (Cobbler pose), *upavistha konasana* (Seated Angle pose), preparation for Lotus pose (not the Full or Half Lotus poses themselves) taking care that you are moving from the hips, lying with legs up the wall, as in *salamba sarvangasana* (Shoulder-stand) against the wall.
See also Arthritis (knees).

L

Laryngitis: *salamba sirsasana* (Head-stand), *adho mukha vrksasana* (Full Arm-balance), *salamba sarvangasana* (Shoulder-stand), *setu bandha sarvangasana* (Bridge pose).

Legs, weakness, aching, strained: all standing postures, followed by *virasana* (Hero pose) and *supta virasana, baddha konasana* (Cobbler pose), *janu sirsasana* (Forward Bend over each Leg), *paschimottanasana* (Sitting Forward Bend), *svanasana* (Dog poses).
See also Varicose veins.

Leukaemia: *salamba sirsasana* (Head-stand), *salamba sarvangasana* (Shoulder-stand) supported, *paschimottanasana* (Sitting Forward Bend) with head resting on block or cushion.

Liver problems: all standing postures, especially *trikonasana* (Triangle pose) and *virabhadrasana I* (first Warrior pose), *janu sirsasana* (Forward Bend over each Leg), *supta virasana*, all back bends, especially *urdhva dhanurasana* (Face-up Bow pose or Back Arch), all twists, especially *jathara parivartanasana* (Lying-down Twist of the Belly). Relaxation, meditation.
See also Hepatitis.

Lung problems: all back bends, *supta virasana, baddha konasana* (Cobbler pose), *bharadvajasana I* (Mermaid pose). Relaxation, *pranayama*.

Lymph problems: all twists, *salamba sarvangasana* (Shoulder-stand)

M

Menopause: *supta virasana* (at least five minutes), *urdhva dhanurasana* (Face-up Bow Pose or Back Arch) over a chair for ten minutes, *supta baddha konasana* (Cobbler pose lying down) for ten minutes; all forward bends. Relaxation, meditation.

Menstrual problems:
Pre-menstrual tension: (to be practised throughout the month but not during or immediately before period:) *salamba sirsasana* (Head-stand), *salamba sarvangasana* (Shoulder-stand), and all back bends; (during period:) *supta virasana* and all forward bends.

Irregularity and pain during period: *supta virasana, svanasana* (Face-up and Face-down Dog poses); all forward bends.

Migraine (at threat of onset): *salamba sirsasana* (Head-stand) between two chairs (right-hand photo on p. 123), *salamba sarvangasana* (Shoulder-stand), all twists especially *jathara parivartanasana* (Lying-down Twist of the Belly), *paschimottanasana* (Sitting Forward Bend) with head on a block or cushion (photo, p. 111), *siddhasana, padmasana* (Full Lotus pose). Relaxation and *pranayama*.
See also Headaches.

Multiple Sclerosis (M.S.): all postures which open the diaphragm out, such as *supta virasana, urdhva dhanurasana* (Face-up Bow pose or Back Arch) over a chair, *baddha konasana*

(Cobbler pose) against the wall, *dandasana* (Staff pose) with hands a little behind the hips so the front of the body opens out more, *upavistha konasana* (Seated Angle pose), *setu bandha sarvangasana* (Bridge pose); where possible, standing postures with back flat against the wall and with a chair to the side to stretch onto.

Myalgic Encephalomyelitis (M.E.): standing postures with back flat against a wall, *salamba sarvangasana* (Shoulder-stand) using wall, chair or blocks where helpful and needed so that you can stay there for five to ten minutes; *setu bandha sarvangasana* (Bridge pose) with support of stool or two or three blocks under sacrum so that you can stay there comfortably for ten to fifteen minutes; *supta virasana, siddhasana.* Relaxation, *pranayama,* meditation.

N

Nausea: *supta virasana, savasana* and *pranayama.*

Neck problems: *salamba sirsasana* (Head-stand) with head between two chairs (photo, p. 123), *adho mukha vrkasana* (Full Arm-balance), in both these postures let head stretch and relax down to ground to relieve neck; *salamba sarvangasana* (Shoulder-stand) with folded blanket or blocks under upper arms *only* as shown in the photo on p. 126; make sure blanket or blocks are high enough to release any pressure on neck. Also, *salamba sarvangasana* on chair is very beneficia; *setu bandha sarvangasana* (Bridge pose), with blanket under upper arms and/or support under sacrum if you feel heavy on the neck; standing postures and twists, concentrating on turning the upper back (*not* the head).

Nervous tension and breakdown: *salamba sirsasana* (Head-stand) and *salamba sarvangasana* (Shoulder-stand) for as long as possible, spending the same time on each; build up to fifteen to twenty minutes on each posture; *svanasana* Face-down Dog pose, *paschimottanasana* (Sitting Forward Bend) with head on block (photo, p. 111) for five to fifteen minutes, *siddhasana, padmasana* (Full Lotus pose). Relaxation, *pranayama,* meditation with

the affirmation 'I am peace, I see peace everywhere'.

Neuralgia: *supta virasana, svanasana* (Face-up and Face-down Dog poses), *baddha konasana* (Cobbler pose), *siddhasana, padmasana* (Full Lotus pose), relaxation, *pranayama,* meditation.

O

Obesity (overweight): *salamba sarvangasana* (Shoulder-stand) for ten to fifteen minutes to adjust thyroid gland, with support where needed; *Surya Namaskar* (Salutation to the Sun). Meditation with the affirmation 'I do not need this weight for protection, it is safe for me to lose weight, to be slim'.

P

Piles: see Haemorrhoids

Polio: (see also handicapped section) standing postures against wall with help, or on floor where possible.

R

Rheumatism and Rheumatoid Arthritis: *svanasana* (Face-up and Face-down Dog poses); standing postures with back flat against wall; *supta virasana, urdhva dhanurasana* (Face-up Bow pose or Back Arch) over a chair.

S

Sciatica: *utthita trikonasana* (Triangle pose) and *utthita parsvakonasana* (Stretched-flank pose) with back against wall; *parsvottanasana, prasarita padottansasana* (Wide Leg-stretch Forward Bend) and *uttanasana* (Standing Forward Bend) with hands on a chair see p. 91; *urdhva dhanurasana* (Face-up Bow pose or Back Arch) starting over a chair and then from floor; *virasana* (Hero pose), *janu sirsasana* (Forward Bend over each Leg) and *upavistha konasana* (Seated Angle pose) both stretching up high with a belt around the feet (do not go forwards), *baddha konasana* (Cobbler pose), *siddhasana, padmasana* (Full Lotus pose). Relaxation with legs on a chair.

Scoliosis: standing postures, *svanasana* (Face-up and Face-down Dog poses); all back bends and all twists. Relaxation on pleated blanket (see photo, p. 166).

Shoulders, tension, aching, strain: all standing postures concentrating on opening chest out, *adho mukha vrksasana* (Full Arm-balance), *svanasana* (Face-up and Face-down Dog poses), all back bends and twists. Relaxation with lift under upper back, so that shoulders can relax down either side.

Round shoulders: standing postures especially *parsvottanasana*, concentrating on opening chest in all these postures; back bends; twists; *supta virasana*, *svanasana* (Face-up and Face-down Dog poses).

Sinus problems: *uttanasana* (Standing Forward Bend), *salamba sarvangasana* (Shoulder-stand), *setu bandha sarvangasana* (Bridge pose), *paschimottanasana* (Sitting Forward Bend). Relaxation, *pranayama* with head lifted on a block.

Spinal problems, disc lesions: all standing postures, *svanasana* (Face-up and Face-down Dog poses), *uttanasana* (Standing Forward Bend), *parsvottanasana*, *prasarita padottanasana* (Wide Leg-stretch Forward Bend), all in the versions with hands on a chair. *No* forward bends. Relaxation with legs on a chair.
See also Back problems, Arthritis, Spine, Scoliosis.

Stomach problems: *svanasana* (Face-up and Face-down Dog poses), *supta virasana*, *jathara parivartanasana* (Lying-down Twist of the Belly), *ardha matsyendrasana I* ('Lord of the Fishes'

pose). Relaxation with legs on a chair.
See also Indigestion Nausea, Heartburn.

Stroke: relaxation, *pranayama*, meditation.

T

Throat problems: *salamba sarvangasana* (Shoulder-stand), *setu bandha sarvangasana* (Bridge pose), *supta virasana*; twists.
See also Colds, Laryngitis.

Tinnitus: *salamba sirsasana* (Head-stand) on two chairs (photo, p. 123); *salamba sarvangasana* (Shoulder-stand) over a chair (photo, p. 127); back bends over a chair, especially *urdhva dhanurasana* (Face-up Bow pose or Back Arch); *supta baddha konasana* (Cobbler pose, lying-down version), *supta virasana*. Meditation.

Thyroid problems: see Throat; Obesity

U

Ulcers: all inverted postures, *jathara parivartanasana* (Lying-down Twist of the Belly), *supta virasana*, *baddha konasana* (Cobbler pose). Relaxation with legs on a chair, *pranayama*, meditation.

V

Varicose Veins: all inverted postures and *svanasana* (Face-up and Face-down Dog poses), followed by *virasana* (Hero pose); *baddha konasana* (Cobbler pose), *upavistha konasana* (Seated Angle pose). Relaxation with legs up the wall or on a chair.

Bibliography

This list includes books mentioned in the text and for further reading, and practice tapes.

White Eagle publications

Grace Cooke, *The Jewel in the Lotus*, Liss, Hants. (The White Eagle Publishing Trust), 1958
—, *Meditation*, Liss, Hants. (The White Eagle Publishing Trust), 1955
—, *Sun Men of the Americas*, Liss, Hants. (The White Eagle Publishing Trust), 1975

Joan Hodgson, *A White Eagle Lodge Book of Health and Healing*, Liss, Hants. (The White Eagle Publishing Trust), 1983
—, *The Stars and the Chakras* (forthcoming) Liss, Hants. (The White Eagle Publishing Trust), 1990
—, *Planetary Harmonies*, Liss, Hants. (The White Eagle Publishing Trust), 1980

White Eagle, *The Gentle Brother*, Liss, Hants. (The White Eagle Publishing Trust), 1968
—, *Golden Harvest*, Liss, Hants. (The White Eagle Publishing Trust), 1958
—, *Prayer in the New Age*, Liss, Hants. (The White Eagle Publishing Trust), 1978
—, *The Quiet Mind*, Liss, Hants. (The White Eagle Publishing Trust), 1972
—, *Spiritual Unfoldment 1*, Liss, Hants. (The White Eagle Publishing Trust), 1961
—, *The Still Voice: a White Eagle Book of Meditation*, Liss, Hants. (The White Eagle Publishing Trust), 1981
—, *The Living Word of St John*, Liss, Hants. (The White Eagle Publishing Trust), 1979

Yoga Practice Tapes

Jenny Beeken, *A First Yoga Practice Tape* CSY01, Liss, Hants. (The White Eagle Publishing Trust)
—, *A Second Yoga Practice Tape* CSY02, Liss, Hants. (The White Eagle Publishing Trust)
—, *Salute to the Sun: A Third Yoga Practice Tape* CSY03, Liss, Hants. (The White Eagle Publishing Trust)
—, *Yoga in Pregnancy: A Fourth Yoga Practice Tape* CSY04, Liss, Hants. (The White Eagle Publishing Trust)

Books by B. K. S. Iyengar

Light on Yoga, London (Unwin Paperbacks), 1966
Light on Pranayama, London (Unwin Paperbacks), 1981
The Tree of Yoga, Oxford (Fine Line Books), 1988

Other Books

[—] *A Course in Miracles*, Tiburon, Calif., (Foundation for Inner Peace), 1975; London (Arkana Books), 1985
Don Aslett, *Freedom from Clutter*, Watford (Exley Publications Ltd), 1985
Richard Bach, *Illusions: the Adventures of a Reluctant Messiah*, London (Pan Books), 1978
J. Allen Boone, *Kinship with all Life*, New York (Harper & Row), 1954

Barbara Brosnan, *Yoga for the Handicapped*, London (Souvenir Press), 1982

Emmanuel's Book: A Manual for Living comfortably in the Cosmos, compiled by Pat Rodegast and Judith Stanton, New York (Bantam Books), 1985

Emmanuel's Book II: The Choice for Love, compiled by Pat Rodegast and Judith Stanton, New York (Bantam Books), 1989

Shakti Gawain, with Laurel King, *Living in the Light: A Guide to Personal and Planetary Transformation*, San Rafael, Calif., (Whatever Publications, Inc.), 1986; London (Eden Grove Editions), 1988

The Geeta: the Gospel of the Lord Shree Krishna, trans. Shree Purohit Swami, London (Faber & Faber), 1935

Gene Gendlin, *Focussing*, New York (Bantam Books), 1983

Susan Hayward, *A Guide for the Advanced Soul*, Crow's Nest, New South Wales (In-Tune Books), 1985

Geeta Iyengar, *Yoga: A Gem for Women*, India (Allied Publishers, Ltd), 1983

Gerald G. Jampolsky, M.D., *Love is Letting Go of Fear*, Berkeley, Calif. (Celestial Arts), 1979

J. K. Krishnamurti, *Krishnamurti's Journal*, London (Victor Gollancz), 1982

F. Leboyer, *The Art of Breathing*, Shaftesbury (Element Books), 1985

F. Leboyer, *Birth without Violence*, Glasgow (Collins Fontana), 1977

F. Leboyer, *Inner Beauty, Inner Light*, Glasgow (Collins Fontana), 1979

Patanjali, *How to Know God: the Yoga Aphorisms of Patanjali*, trans. with commentary by Swami Prabhavananda and Christopher Isherwood, New York (New American Library), 1969

Sondra Ray, *The Only Diet There is*, Berkeley, Calif. (Celestial Arts), 1981

Sondra Ray, *Loving Relationships*, Berkeley, Calif. (Celestial Arts), 1980

The Upanishads, trans. Alistair Shearer and Peter Russell, London (Unwin Paperbacks), 1989

The Upanishads, trans. Juan Mascaró, London (Penguin Books), 1965

Paramahansa Yogananda, *Autobiography of a Yogi*, London (Rider), revised edn., 1987

Useful Addresses

The White Eagle Lodge, New Lands, Brewells Lane, Liss, Hampshire, England, GU33 7HY (tel. 0730 893300)

The White Eagle Lodge, 9 St Mary Abbots Place, Kensington, London W8 6LS (tel. 071-603 7914)

Church of the White Eagle Lodge, P. O. Box 930, Montgomery, Texas, 77356, U.S.A. (tel. 409 597 5757)

The White Eagle Lodge (Australasia), P. O. Box 225, Maleny, Queensland 4552 (tel. 71 944397)

The Iyengar Yoga Institute, 223a Randolph Avenue, London W9 (tel. 071-624 3080)

Yoga for Health Foundation, Ickwell Bury, Biggleswade, Beds. (tel. 0491 39489)

The Dr Edward Bach Centre, Mount Vernon, Sotwell, Wallingford, Oxon. OX10 0PZ (tel. 076727 271)

The Gerda Boyesen Centre, Acacia House, Centre Avenue, Acton Park, London W3 7JX (tel. 081-743 2437) (for Bioenergetics)

Universal Training (formerly The Self-Transformation Centre), Tempo House, Suite 35, 15 Falcon Road, Battersea, London SW11 2PJ (tel. 071-223 7662)

Jenny Beeken, c/o The White Eagle Lodge, New Lands (see above)

Index to the Postures